THE ROYAL LIFE SAVING SOCIETY

★ *Swim*

Survive ★

★ *Save*

THE ROYAL LIFE SAVING SOCIETY

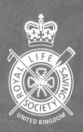

ROYAL LIFE SAVING SOCIETY

UNITED KINGDOM

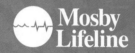

Mosby
Lifeline

St. Louis Baltimore Boston Carlsbad Chicago Naples New York Philadelphia Portland

London Madrid Mexico City Singapore Sydney Tokyo Toronto Wiesbaden

Swim ★ Survive ★ Save

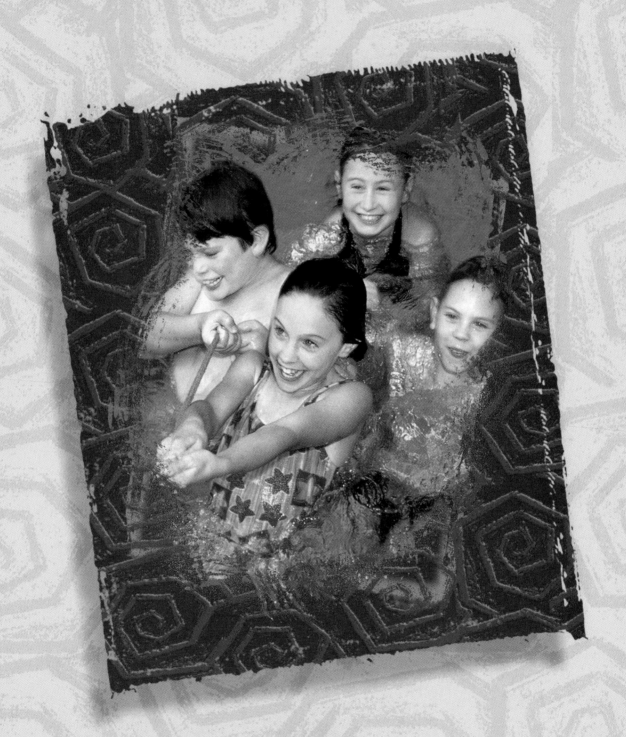

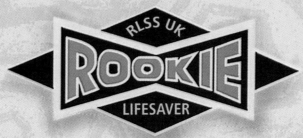

RLSS UK
ROOKIE
LIFESAVER

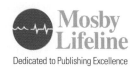
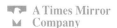

Dedicated to Publishing Excellence

A Times Mirror
Company

Senior Vice President & Publisher: John A. Hirst
Author: Peter Banham
Vice President, Editing, Design & Production: Robert Passantino
Book Design: Studio Montage
Photography: Tim Fisher, Gary Otte
Editorial Development Board: David Axam, Pauline Cox, David Eaton,
   Lisbeth Jensen, George Toft

Composition by Studio Montage, St. Louis, U.S.A.

Printing and binding by Donnelley Bright Sun Printing Co. Ltd.

ISBN 0-7234-2768-2

Acknowledgements

First a big thanks to the Rookies who we follow throughout this book. They did a marvellous job, repeating the skills and spending hours in the pool. Thanks to Sophie Jones, Alice Felstead, Sam Dalglish, Matthew Blaiklock, Jo McCarthy, Amelia Sayell, Christopher Buckmaster, Pia Conchie, Andrew Roberts and Natasha Parmar.

Thanks to: Sarah Morrell, Leon Duhaney, Thorunn Larusdoltir, Ian Ware, Antony Penge, Fiona Alderman, Pauline Dalglish, Peter Dalglish, Alan Percival, Lisbeth Jensen, Bert Vander Mark, Jan McCarthy, Rebekah Wilson, Emma-Jane Rose, Peter Banham, Caroline Larby, Annette Martin, Adrian Attwell, Linda Painter, Ann Dewar, Jane Ellison, Sam Ellison, Billy Ellison, Barry Taylor for playing different parts in the photos and Paul King.

Thanks also go to the following for loan of equipment: Keith, Johnson and Pelling Ltd., Terry Upperdine, Rushmoor Voluntary Lifeguards, Alan Percival, Kingfisher Leisure Center and Nikon for lending us an underwater camera.

The pool photos were taken at the Kingfisher Leisure Centre, Kingston-upon-Thames and The Spectrum, Guildford. Some indoor shots were taken at Cafe Select at The Spectrum, Guildford.

Thanks to Surrey Ambulance Service for lending us an ambulance and, especially to the two paramedics Lisa Selby and Roz Holder from Chertsey ambulance station.

External review provided by the editorial board consisting of: George Toft (RLSS UK), Pauline Cox (RLSS UK), Keith Holman (SLSA GB), David Eaton (Education and Technical Committee), Stephen Lear (Director), David Axam (Chairman, Promotions Committee) and Lisbeth Jensen (Rookie Youth Development Officer). Technical review and support was provided by Dr. A J Handley (RLSS UK President and Chief Medical Advisor), Olive Bowes (Chairman RLSS UK Education and Technical Committee and the Editorial Board).

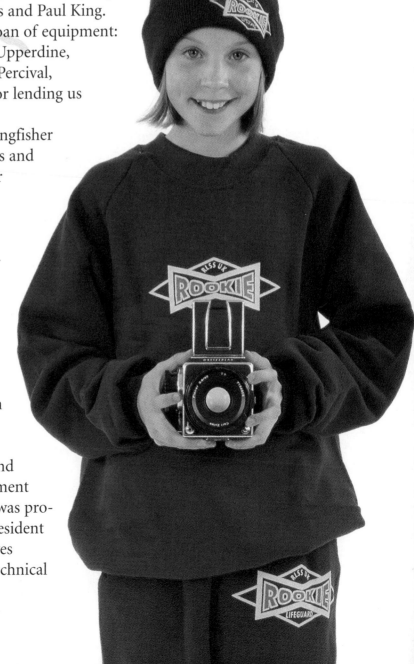

The following are acknowledged for lending photographs: Surrey Ambulance Service for the photo of a emergency dispatch room on page 9. Callum Farquhar for the photo of a Scottish Loch on page 13. The Shropshire Star for the photo of a car in the water on page 27. The RNLI for the picture of a lifeboat on page 10. HM Coastguard for the photo of a HM Coastguard helicopter on page 10. The Royal Life Saving Society Australia for the use of the illustration and photo of a rip current on page 92, the illustration of different types of waves on page 91, the illustrations of swimming in waves on page 91, illustrations of standing from floating on page 34, the sculling hands on page 36, the illustrations of two sinking cars on page 27 and the illustrations of removing clothes on page 51. The Canadian Red Cross Society for the picture of getting into a boat on page 22 and Gary Otte for the photo of a man in the ice on page 24. The American Red Cross for the three pictures of visibility in water on page 21.

Much support and help has been received from all the staff at RLSS UK Headquarters at Mountbatten House and Mosby Lifeline. At Mosby Lifeline especially Fiona Alderman and John Hirst have been very supportive.

Special thanks to all the staff at Studio Montage for design and electronic production, Peter Banham—Lifesaving Development Manager for writing a comprehensive technical manuscript, Jackie Roberts for editing and Tim Fisher for photography where nothing else is credited.

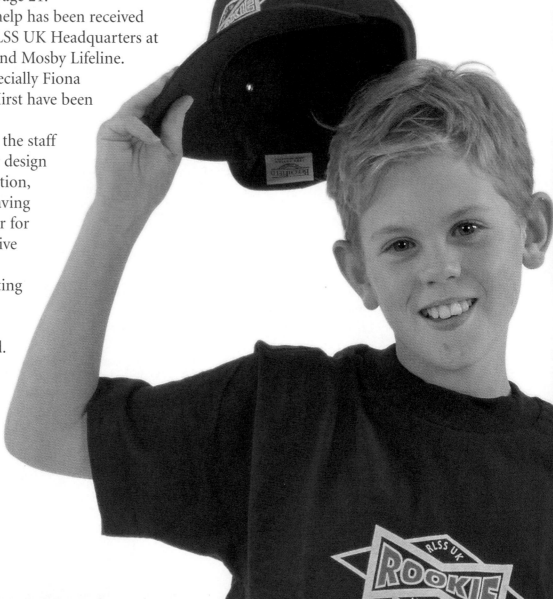

Introduction

Hi! My name is Sarah and this is my friend Leon. We are both Lifeguards with the Royal Life Saving Society UK. We are going to tell you how to use this book so you will have fun and get the best out of it.

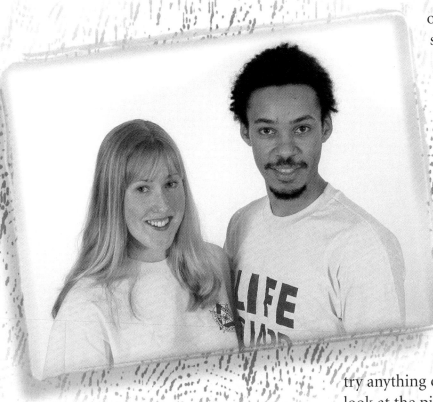

In the book you will find out about all the different swimming, survival and lifesaving skills Rookies need to know. You can join a Rookie course at your local swimming pool or take the book with you to the pool and try out some of the skills with your friends. The book is full of photographs of some of our Rookie friends. The ten Rookies featured will show you how you can learn to carry out these lifesaving skills yourself. So before you try anything out in the pool have a good look at the pictures and read all about them.

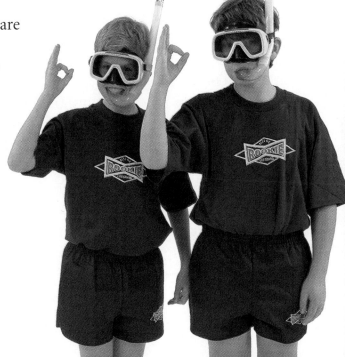

Make sure you tell the pool lifeguard what you are planning to do before you try out any lifesaving skills. It is always a good idea to have a grown-up watching you in the water especially when you are trying out some of the more difficult skills. You never know what will happen, especially the first time!

Look out for some special symbols as you read the book. If you see a half-filled square ▱ next to a practice, it means you should do it in shallow water. If you see a square that is filled in ■, it means you should practise in deep water. **Shallow water is less than 1.5 metres deep and deep water is more than 1.5 metres deep.** Make sure you stick to this as it will keep you safe in the water.

As you read the book you will also see lots of Rookie Tips. These are special hints that we think will help you carry out the rescue skills really well or tips we think you should know.

Each chapter of this book follows the Rookie Programme. There is a chapter on Water Safety, Self Rescue, Rescue and Emergency Response. The final chapter is about sea awareness, equipment, snorkelling, paddle craft and communications. To make them easy for you to follow, we have divided Chapters 2, 3 and 5 into two parts.

The first part tells you about what is in the chapter. The second part, called "Now You Try It!", shows you how to do the skills. You can practise these skills in the pool with your friends. We have made sure there are plenty of photographs, all you need to do is open the page and copy what you see.

In Chapter 4 you can learn about CPR and Rescue Breathing. If you try this remember that the CPR and Rescue Breathing techniques described should only be practised on a resuscitation manikin—never on a living person.

We are sure you will enjoy learning all these important skills with your friends. Don't forget they are really useful and one day may help you to save someone's life.

The Rookie Programme

The RLSS UK Rookie Programme is great fun and if you are aged between 5 and 13, it has been designed specifically for YOU.

If you become a Rookie, you will learn special lifesaving skills to help save yourself and others who get into difficulty in the water. You will also learn what you can do if somebody stops breathing or if someone's heart stops beating.

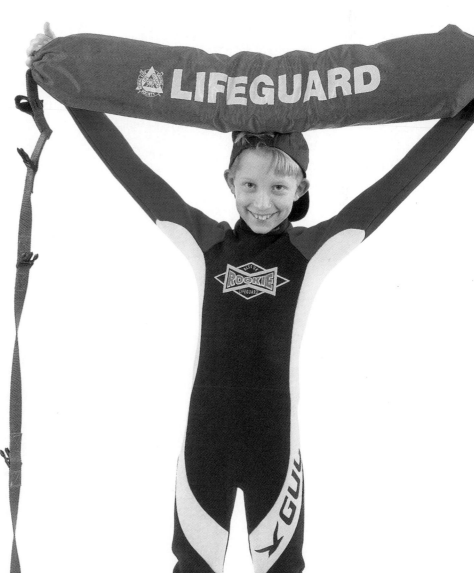

The Rookie Programme has four main sections:

Water Safety where you learn how to stay safe and keep others safe near water.

Self Rescue where you learn how to survive in water and help yourself if you get into difficulties.

Rescue where you learn when and how to rescue people in trouble.

Emergency Response where you learn what to do to help someone who has stopped breathing or has no pulse and how to keep them alive until help arrives.

There are also five other sections about lifeguarding. These are extras and you do not have to do them.

Sea Awareness explains about the sea, waves and currents.

Equipment is about the equipment, such as torpedo buoys and throw bags which lifeguards use to rescue people.

Snorkelling shows you how to use mask, snorkel and fins.

Paddle Craft is about how to use body boards, rescue skis and rescue boards to make rescues.

Communications teaches you the signals used by lifeguards and how to pass on information.

If you join Rookie you will be learning in a swimming pool not in a classroom. You will have fun with your friends and learn many new skills. It is very easy to join—all you need is a swimming costume and a towel.

The Rookie Programme is divided into 4 Star Grades which are split up into 4 levels. There are lots of achievement badges and certificates for you to work towards. You do not always need to start on Star Grade One Level One, you can start higher up if you have already received some training. Check with your Rookie Trainer about this.

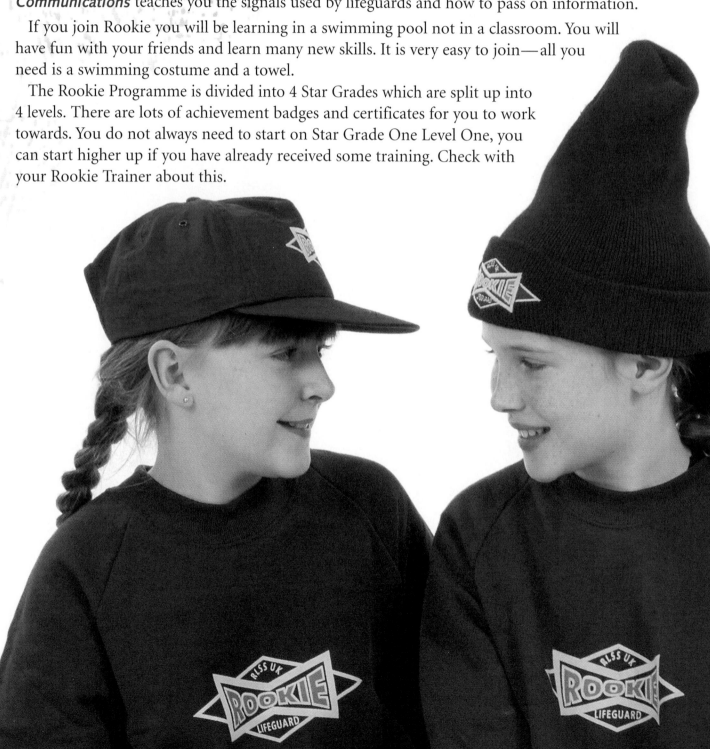

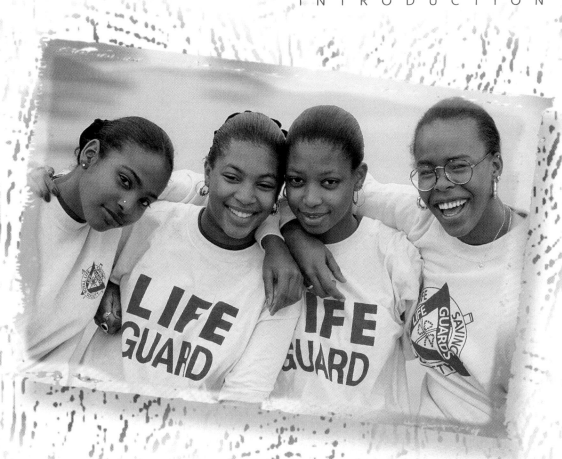

You can buy all the equipment you need to take part in the programme from RLSS UK Enterprises Ltd. You can also buy Rookie T-shirts, sweatshirts, jogging bottoms, hats, mask, snorkel and fins. Ask your Rookie Trainer for a Rookie Catalogue or contact RLSS UK Enterprises Ltd at the address you will find at the back of this book.

How to Join

If you would like to become a Rookie you should first ask at your local swimming pool or Leisure Centre if the programme is run there. If it is not, then you should contact the RLSS UK at the address at the back of this book. They can help you find out more.

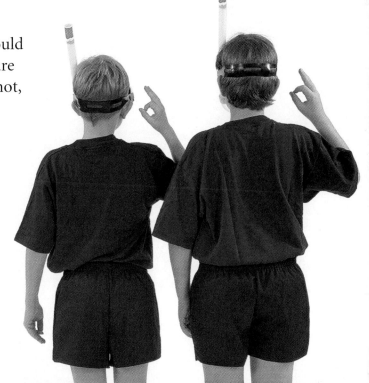

Table of Contents

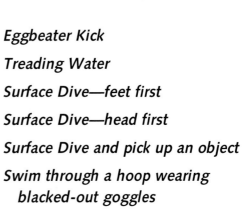

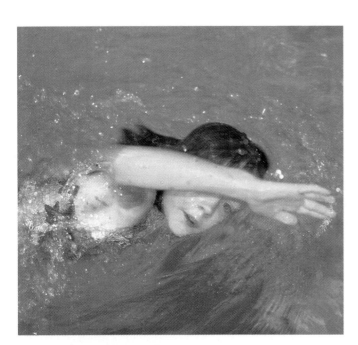

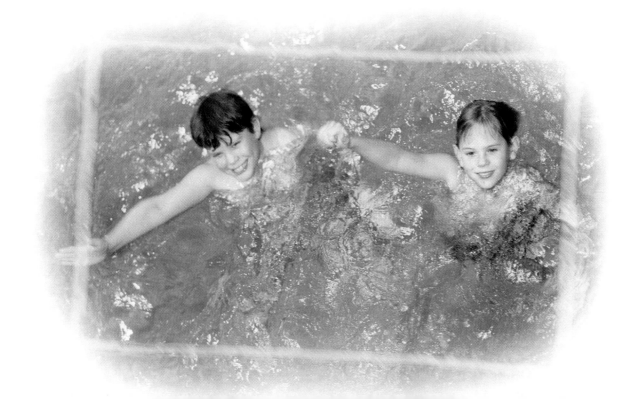

Chapter 3
Rescue

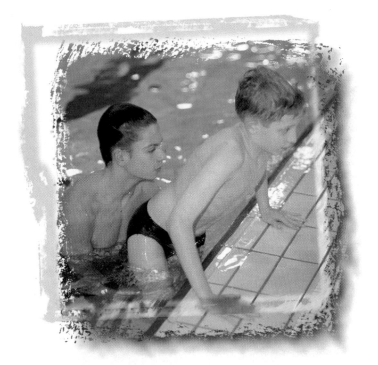

Chapter 4
Emergency Response

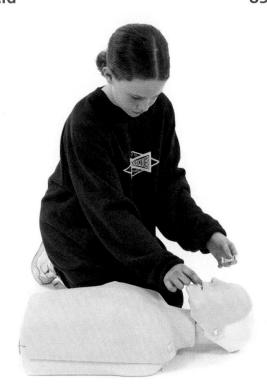

Chapter 5
Lifeguarding and Equipment Skills

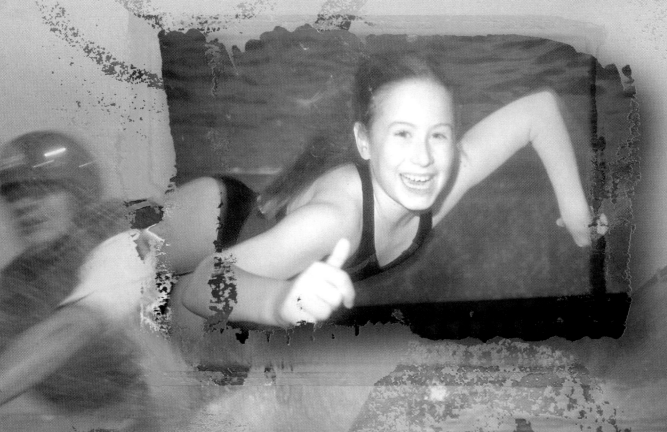

Water Safety

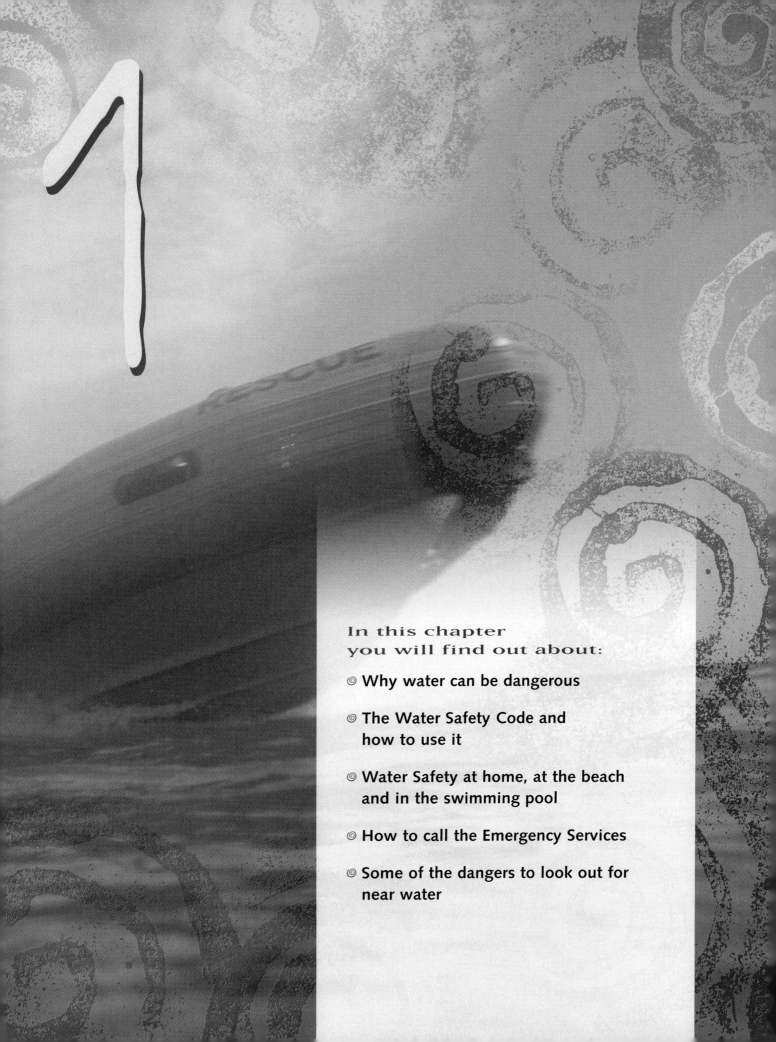

1

In this chapter you will find out about:

- Why water can be dangerous

- The Water Safety Code and how to use it

- Water Safety at home, at the beach and in the swimming pool

- How to call the Emergency Services

- Some of the dangers to look out for near water

It is great fun to be near the water – there is always lots to do. Water can also be very dangerous and you need to know how to avoid possible dangers.

WHY IS WATER DANGEROUS?

Water is dangerous because it can kill you. You need to breathe in air all the time so that you will stay alive. If you block off the air supply, you can die. You may drown if you hold your nose and mouth under the water for any length of time, unless of course you have got a snorkel or a tank of compressed air such as divers use.

People drown in many different places including swimming pools, ponds, rivers, the sea and even in the bath. The water doesn't have to be very deep. Every year a number of very young children drown in places with only a few inches of water such as puddles, buckets, baths and garden ponds. (See page 11.)

Don't think that because you are a good swimmer you won't get into difficulties. Strong swimmers often drown because they are not really as good as they think they are and because they don't realise how severe the danger is. Rookies must always be aware of the possible hazards.

Remember to empty buckets when you have finished with them

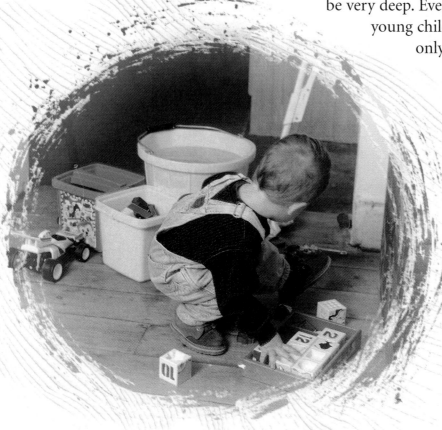

Drownings in Britain

Each year about 500 people in Britain drown.
The places where you are most likely
to drown are in rivers, streams,
lakes, reservoirs, canals and the
sea. These are places that are
normally unsupervised. These
are also places where the water
is murky and where it is difficult
to see the bottom or how deep it
is. The water is usually cold, with
hidden currents and underwater
obstacles. The depth may change suddenly
and swimmers can find it difficult or impossible to climb out.

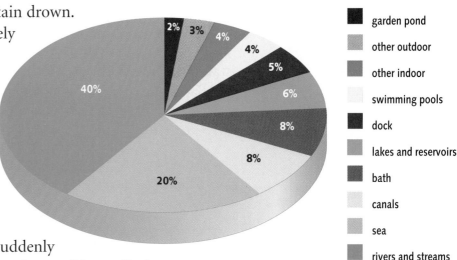

Places people drown

- garden pond
- other outdoor
- other indoor
- swimming pools
- dock
- lakes and reservoirs
- bath
- canals
- sea
- rivers and streams

THE WATER SAFETY CODE

Whenever you are near water, you
should follow the Water Safety Code.

1 Spot The Dangers

Whenever you are around water
always take extra care. Look out for
possible dangers—you may be able
to prevent accidents before they
happen. If you spot anything in or
beside the water which could be
dangerous, you should report it
immediately. Tell someone in charge,
such as a lifeguard, lock keeper or
a farmer. You can also fill in a
Rookie Community Response
Form and send to whoever is in
charge—perhaps the local council
or police. This way whatever you
have spotted will get fixed much
more quickly.

Things to look out for:

- missing rescue equipment
- a damaged warning sign
  or fence
- a broken public telephone.

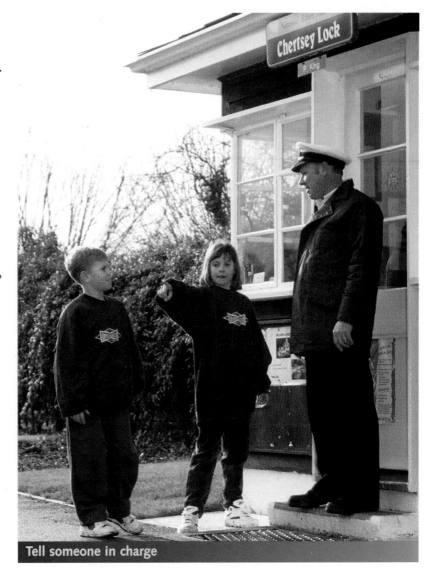

Tell someone in charge

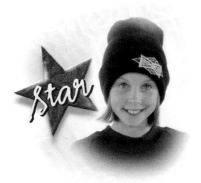

Rookie

Hi, my name is Sophie and I go to St John's Primary School and my hobbies are swimming, dancing and Rookie. Rookie is fun and I learn lifesaving skills that I can use to help other people.

Remember what you do could save someone's life. You can get the Rookie Community Response Forms from your Trainer or RLSS UK and keep them in your Rookie Logbook. When you hand one in, make a copy to keep for yourself.

Don't forget that accidents may be caused by the way in which you and your friends behave.

- Never fool around or run by the water—you could trip and fall in.
- Take care on the riverbank— it may be slippery or it could crumble away.
- Keep well away from the canal edge— the water is usually very deep.
- Beware of locks and weirs— the water flows very quickly.
- Stay right away from gravel pits.
- Take care near flooded areas and polluted water.
- Keep away from canal locks unless you are in a boat.
- Only swim in open water if there is a grown-up in charge.

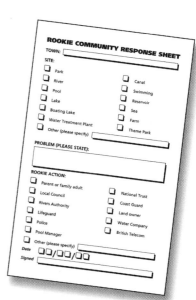

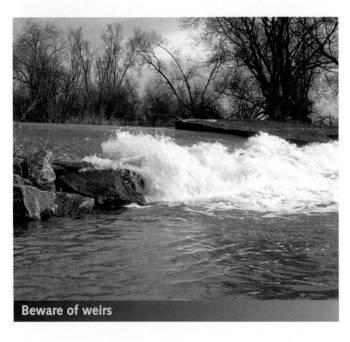

Beware of weirs

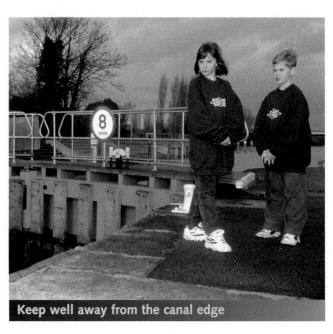

Keep well away from the canal edge

- Don't stand on overhanging, sloping, slippery rocks or banks.
- Avoid diving in—but if you have to, only dive in where you can see the bottom to make sure it is deep enough. Never dive into water less than 1.5 metres deep.

Some Warning Signs...

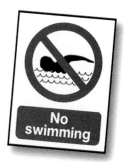

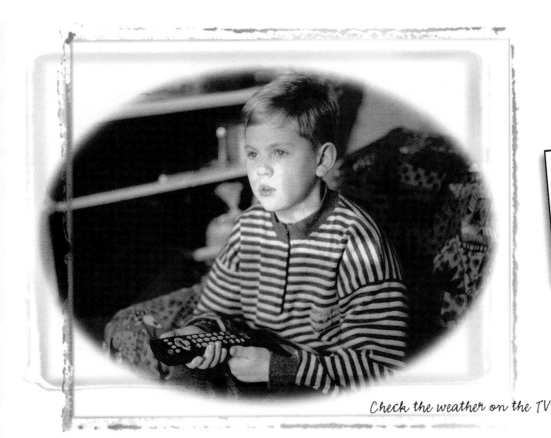

Check the weather on the TV

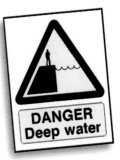

❷ Take Safety Advice

Before you go into the water, make sure you have found out as much as possible about where you are going. There are a number of ways you can find things out.

- Listen to the weather forecast on the radio or TV, before you go out.
- When you arrive at the beach or pool ask the lifeguard where it is safe to swim.
- Look for warning signs and flags telling you what you can or can't do.
- Ask a grown-up if the water is safe— never swim where it is dangerous.

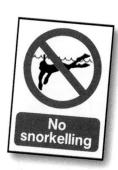

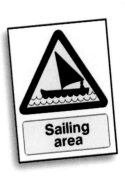

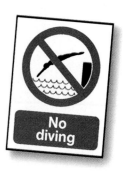

❸ Don't Go Alone

Never go swimming on your own unless you are in a pool with lifeguards to keep an eye on you. If you do get into difficulties, there may be nobody to help you. Stay safe and always swim with someone else. Remember it is always best if there is a lifeguard on duty.

Always tell a grown-up where you are going and when you will be back. If you go with someone else they can telephone or go for help, even if they can't rescue you themselves.

❹ Learn How To Help

Learning how to help means knowing how to help yourself and other people when something goes wrong. The main things you need to know are in Chapter 2—Self Rescue (helping yourself), Chapter 3—Rescue (helping others), and Chapter 4—Emergency Response (helping others).

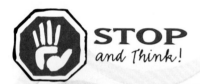

STOP *and Think!*

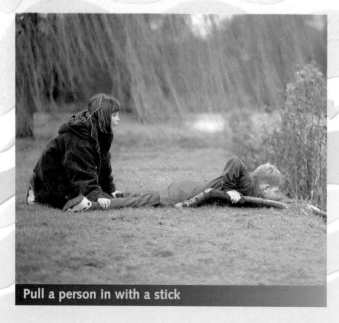

Pull a person in with a stick

IF YOU DO have to make an emergency rescue, always put your own safety first.

- *Keep calm and think before you do something.*
- *Try to get help by shouting "help, help!" as loudly as you can.*
- *Try and pull the person to land with a stick, pole, towel or a piece of clothing. Lie down to make sure you don't get pulled in too.*
- *If you can't reach the person throw them something that floats.*
- *If no one comes when you shout, run to the nearest house or public telephone and dial 999 and ask for help. (See page 9.)*

Learning how to help is easy. Start by learning how to swim, then train for your Rookie Rescue, Self Rescue and Emergency Response Star Grades.

Learn the Water Safety Code

1 ★ Spot the Danger   3 ★ Don't Go Alone

2 ★ Take Safety Advice   4 ★ Learn How to Help

CALLING THE EMERGENCY SERVICES

In Britain the emergency telephone number is 999. Whenever you are out with your friends, especially if you are near open water, check where the nearest telephone is and make sure it is working.

When You Dial 999

You don't need any money.

- Press or dial 999 slowly.
- Tell the operator which service you want:
    Police
    Fire Brigade
    Coastguard
    Ambulance
    Mountain Rescue
- Tell the operator the telephone number shown on the telephone so he can phone you back if you get cut off.
- Wait for the Emergency Service to answer.
- Give the address or place where help is needed.
- Briefly tell them what has happened. Say how many people are involved and what their condition is.
- Give your name, home address and telephone number if asked.

Rookie Tip: Keep calm and remember to speak clearly and carefully. The operator may need to ask you some questions about what has happened, so try and remember the details.

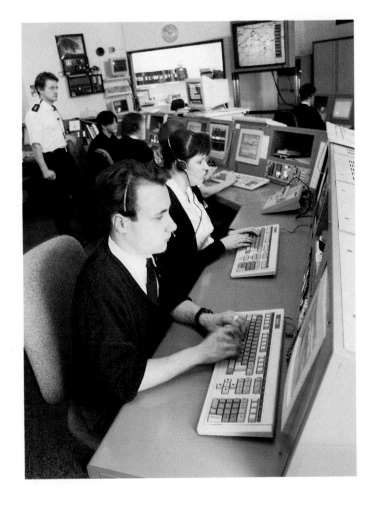

EMERGENCIES AROUND THE COAST

Search and rescue around the coast is managed by HM Coastguard who organises lifeboats, inshore rescue boats and helicopters. If you see an emergency around the coast or in the sea, dial 999 and ask for the Coastguard.

- **Lifeboats** come from the Royal National Lifeboat Institution (RNLI).
- **Inshore Rescue Boats** come from different organisations including the Royal Life Saving Society UK (RLSS UK) and the Surf Life Saving Association of Great Britain (SLSA).
- **Helicopters** come from HM Coastguard, the Royal Navy and the Royal Air Force.

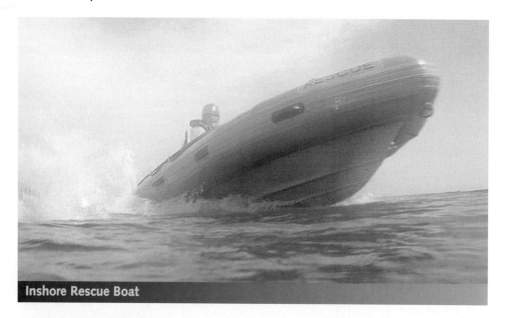

Inshore Rescue Boat

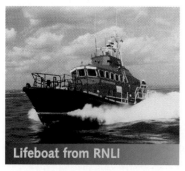

Lifeboat from RNLI

Rookie Tip: If you are in the water yourself, you should not try a rescue but swim to safety and then either get help right away or begin your Rookie Action Plan. (See page 59.)

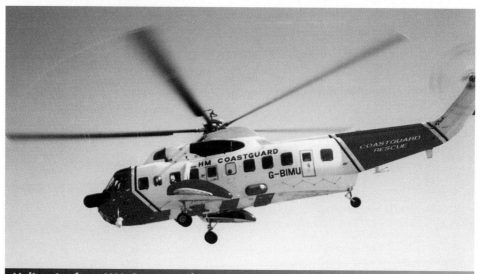

Helicopter from HM Coastguard

WATER SAFETY

At Home

If you have younger brothers or sisters, you should watch out for all the ordinary things that can be dangerous to young children. Paddling pools, washing machines, sinks and baths can all be dangerous if left full of water. Make sure they are emptied as soon as they have been used. In the garden make sure that gates are kept closed, water containers such as water butts are covered, ponds have netting over the top, and swimming pools are covered over. **Remember that young children need someone to keep an eye on them all the time!**

Rookie Tip: Empty paddling pools when you are finished with them.

In the Swimming Pool

When you go to the swimming pool, you should set a good example to others by acting responsibly.

- Listen to the lifeguards.
- Leave the pool if a lifeguard tells you to.
- Read and obey any signs giving advice to swimmers.
- Check the depth markings on the poolside to see where it is best to swim and dive.
- Don't run around the pool.

Outside

Water that you find outside, apart from swimming pools, is called "open water." This is where people are most likely to drown and includes such places as rivers, streams, reservoirs, lakes, canals and the sea. If you see an emergency happening in open water, dial 999 and ask for the police or fire service. Don't forget that although the sea is open water, you should dial 999 and ask for the Coastguard.

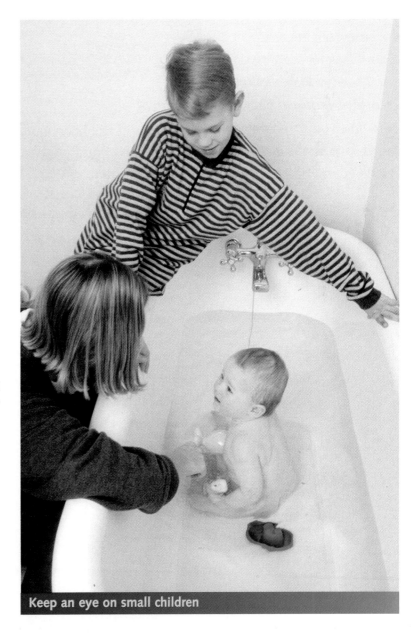

Keep an eye on small children

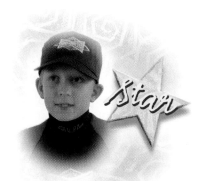

Rookie

*H*i, my name is Chris and I like going to the beach. On the beach I always look for the lifeguard hut. There are lifeguard huts on many beaches in Britain. Next time you are on the beach, look for the lifeguards yourself.

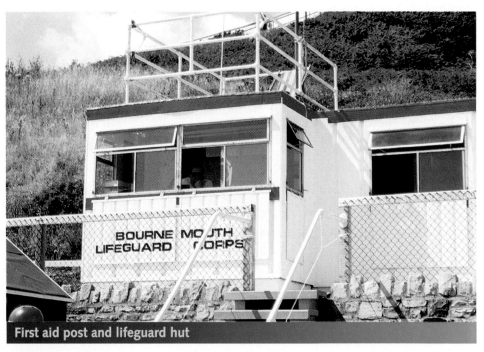

First aid post and lifeguard hut

At the Beach

The water at the beach and seaside can be very dangerous because of tides, waves and currents. (See page 90.)

Stay safe when you are at the sea.

- Look out for warning flags or signs and obey them.
- Find out where and when it is safe to swim and check the tide times.
- Make sure inflatables are tied to the beach by a line.
- Keep out of the way of surfboards and boats.
- Stay in the swimming area and swim parallel to the shore, not further out to sea.
- Notice where the lifeguard, nearest telephone and First Aid post are.
- Get out if you start feeling cold and make sure you know how to signal for help if you need it. (See page 25.)
- Never climb up cliffs or explore caves unless a qualified grown-up is with you.

DANGERS

Alcohol

It is very dangerous to go swimming after drinking alcohol. Alcohol can make you feel as if you don't care about taking risks. Your body loses energy more quickly, you can't swim as well as you usually can and you can soon become cold. Every year people drown because they go swimming when they have been drinking alcohol.

Rookie Tip: Advise your older friends not to drink alcohol and swim!

Cold Water

Open water is much colder than water in a swimming pool. The water in reservoirs, lochs, lakes and rivers is usually very deep, so it never gets the chance to warm up—even during heatwaves. Although it may feel warm around the edges, you will find that if you swim a few metres from the shore, the temperature can suddenly drop, causing **cold shock.** Water cools you much faster than air does. When you are cold, you lose your strength, you move more slowly and you can't swim so far. Many people drown because they don't realise that cold water makes a person weak.

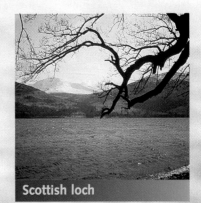
Scottish loch

This is what happens when you fall into cold water:

- The temperature of your skin and your blood drops quickly.
- At first you may gasp for breath and find it difficult to breathe—this is called **cold shock.**
- You find it more and more difficult to move your hands.
- The temperature of your heart, brain and other vital organs falls slowly.
- You start shivering.
- If you stay in the water, you may become unconscious and drown.

Gasping for air, together with the cold shock you feel when you first enter the water, can make you breathe in water, cause a heart attack and you may drown.

Rookie Tip: Never cool off by jumping into open water. Go to the swimming pool instead.

Cold Shock Next time you have a shower, try turning the water temperature to cold and see how you gasp for air. This will give you an idea of what cold shock is like.

One of the other dangers of cold water is **hypothermia.** (See page 83.) This could kill you even after you are out of water.

For further information on survival and what to do on ice, see Chapter 2—Self Rescue.

Sunshine

When the weather is hot, everyone wants to go outside and enjoy the sunshine. Even on a cloudy day, the sun can easily burn you. It is important to protect yourself from the harmful rays of the sun when you are outdoors. To protect yourself put on some sun cream.

Make sure that the sun cream has a Sun Protection Factor that suits your skin. The fairer your skin, the higher the number you need. Ask your local chemist for advice.

Rookies should always be safe under the sun, so **SLIP, SLAP, SLOP!**

Slip, Slap, Slop

Rookie Tip: To protect yourself from the sun, remember to:

- **SLIP** *on a long sleeved T-shirt.*
- **SLAP** *on a broad rimmed hat.*
- **SLOP** *on some sun cream.*

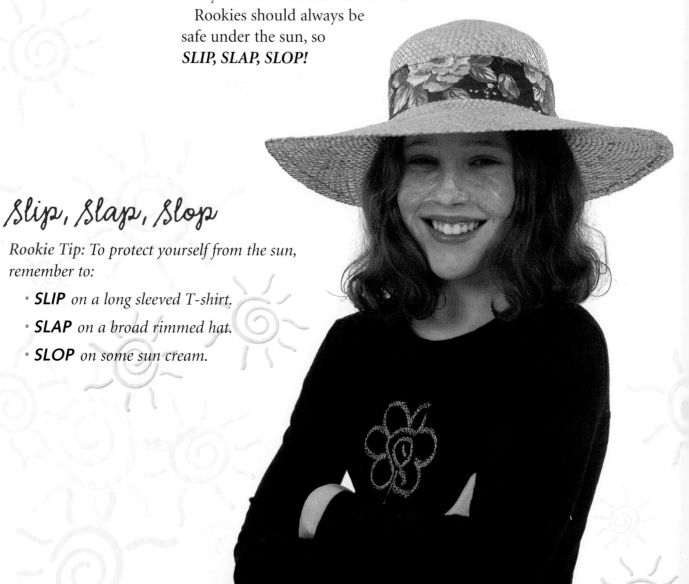

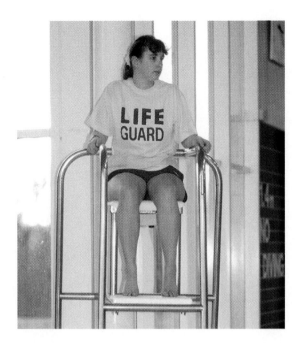

THE LIFEGUARD

A lifeguard is responsible for "guarding" the lives of swimmers in the water. By always being on the look out for problems, the highly trained pool or beach lifeguard can prevent accidents from happening and deal with emergencies. For more information on lifeguards, see page 88.

Rookie Lifeguard Potential

As a Rookie you should show that you have lifeguard potential by learning how to help and by being able and willing to help when needed. (See Chapter 3.) You should always think about your safety and other people's safety when you are in or near the water.

RLSS UK Rookie — Water Safety Certificate

The Rookie Programme includes a Water Safety Certificate for 4 Star Grades. This can be taken either on its own or as part of other Rookie training.

Activities

*T*o learn more about water safety, try some of the following ideas either on your own or with friends.

Water Safety Code

Check out your local swimming pool and see how well you can apply the Water Safety Code.

Spot the Dangers

Draw a picture of a pool, a beach, a lake or a river and in it show as many of the possible dangers that you can think of.

Emergency Services

With your partner pretend that you need to phone for help. Your partner is the telephone operator for the emergency services. Do this by pretending to phone the coastguard, police, ambulance and fire brigade.

Water Safety Outside

Try making an alphabetical list of dangers or emergencies.
For example, *A is for Alcohol . . .*

Slip, Slap, Slop

Try putting a T-shirt, hat and suncream on your partner when you are blindfolded. How quickly can you do it? Take care not to get the suncream in his eyes.

Self Rescue

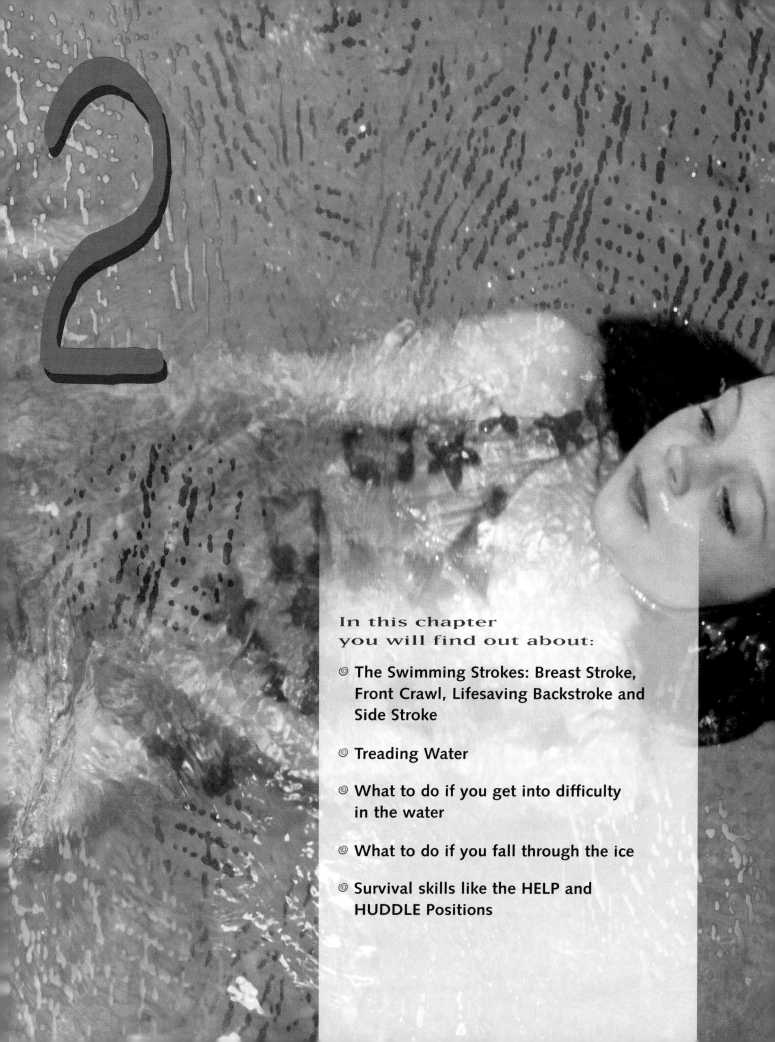

2

In this chapter
you will find out about:

◎ The Swimming Strokes: Breast Stroke,
Front Crawl, Lifesaving Backstroke and
Side Stroke

◎ Treading Water

◎ What to do if you get into difficulty
in the water

◎ What to do if you fall through the ice

◎ Survival skills like the HELP and
HUDDLE Positions

If you get into difficulties when you are in the water, don't panic! There are a number of things you can learn to do to help yourself and to help anyone coming to rescue you. Find out about them in this chapter.

This chapter has two parts. The first part tells you about the skills. The second part, "Now You Try it!" shows you how to practise the skills. Have fun!

Rookie Tip: Tell the lifeguard what you are doing before practising any lifesaving skills.

Before You Get Into The Water

Remember to stop and ask yourself these four questions:

- *How deep is the water?*
- *How high up am I from the water?*
- *Can I see the bottom?*
- *How quickly do I need to get in?*

GETTING INTO THE WATER SAFELY

Slide-in Entry You can get in this way if there are no steps and you can't see what is under the water or don't know how deep it is.

Step-in Entry This is one way of getting in where the water is more than 1.5 metres deep.

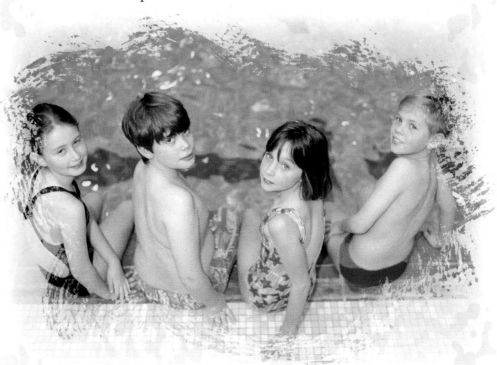

Straddle Entry When you get in this way, your head does not go under the water which is good because you don't lose sight of the casualty. You can use this if the water is more than 1.5 metres deep and you can see the bottom.

Compact Jump Use this when you are standing more than 1 metre above the water.

Diving A Shallow Dive is the quickest way of getting into water that is more than 1.5 metres deep. Make sure you can confidently do a

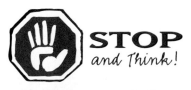

NEVER DIVE into shallow water which is less than 1.5 metres deep or into murky water where you can't see the bottom.

Sitting Dive, a Kneeling Dive and a Lunge Dive before you try a Shallow Dive.

Falling in Sometimes you will get into the water by accident! Remember, if you do fall in, you need to react quickly! Take a big breath and tuck up into a ball before you hit the water. Swim to safety as soon as you come up to the surface.

SWIMMING

Swimming is fun. When you learn how to swim you should begin by learning how to float and scull. When you can do both these things confidently, it is time to learn some of the special swimming strokes. Rookies need to become good swimmers so remember, if you go swimming regularly you will get stronger and be able to swim further.

Floating This is an important thing to learn and it is fun too! Make sure you can stand up safely in the water before you try floating!

Sculling This is a special way of swimming just by moving your hands. This helps you to keep afloat in the water when you are tired.

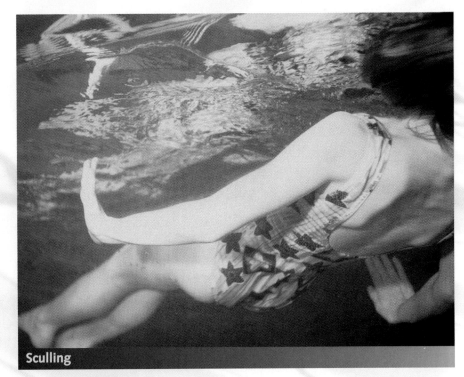

Sculling

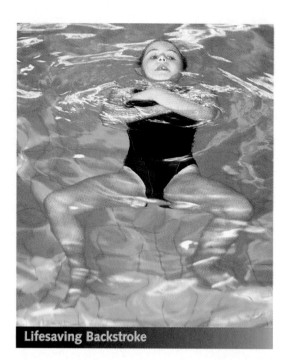

Lifesaving Backstroke

Swimming Strokes When you are swimming, think about these four things:
- The shape of your body
- The way you kick your legs
- How you use your arms
- How you breathe

Lifesavers need to learn Front Crawl, Breast Stroke, Side Stroke and Lifesaving Backstroke so you need to learn how to swim on your front and back. You also need to learn how to change from one stroke to another without stopping and how to swim using just your arms or legs on their own.

Front Crawl This is the fastest stroke because your body is stretched right out in the water and you are using your strong arm and leg muscles at the same time.

Breast Stroke This is a slower stroke and is a good stroke to use if you have a long way to swim. It is useful for lifesaving because you can keep an eye on the casualty as you swim towards him.

Lifesaving Backstroke This stroke will leave you with both hands free to hold the casualty as you swim.

Side Stroke You can use this stroke as you tow someone through the water. As you swim you can see in front of you and behind you.

Eggbeater Kick This may have a funny name but it is the strongest kick for treading water and is also useful when you are towing a casualty.

Treading Water This is swimming "on the spot" because you are staying in one place in deep water. When you can swim on your front and back in deep water, you are ready to learn this very important survival skill.

SWIMMING UNDERWATER

You should practise how to surface dive and swim underwater safely.

Surface Diving

If you want to swim underwater you need to know how to surface dive. There are two ways to do this. Feet first is the safest, so do this when you don't know what is under the water. The other way is head first. This is quicker but should only be done if you can see under the water.

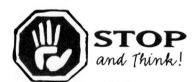

STOP *and Think!*

YOU MUST NEVER attempt to practise surface diving in water more than 1.5 metres deep!

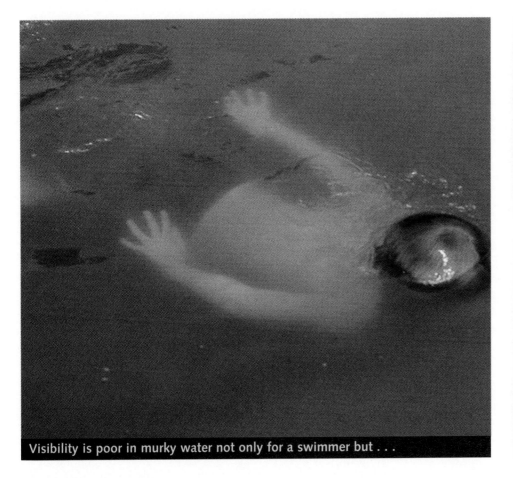

Visibility is poor in murky water not only for a swimmer but . . .

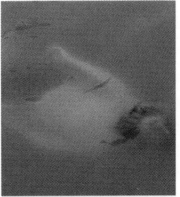

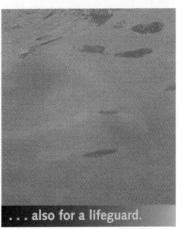

. . . also for a lifeguard.

Finding Your Way Underwater

It is easy to see underwater in the swimming pool but in the sea, lake or river it can be very murky. This means that you will have to feel your way around underwater by touch. For some ideas on how to practise this in the swimming pool. (See page 49.)

Clearing Your Ears

Sometimes going under the water can make your ears hurt. To stop this from happening, use your finger and thumb to pinch your nostrils closed as you go under. At the same time close your mouth and gently try to blow air out through your nose. You should feel your ears go "pop". You should not swim under water if you have problems with your ears, a blocked nose or if you have grommets. If you are not sure, check with your parent or guardian first.

Rookie Tip: If your ears don't pop or if they start to hurt, come up to the surface immediately.

Wading

Wading is walking through shallow water. As you wade through moving water use a pole or stick to feel the bottom in front of you. You will find it easier to keep your balance if you walk with your feet apart and move slowly.

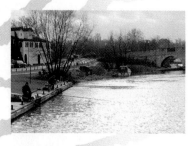

Open Water

There are two types of Open Water.

Moving Water Includes tides at the seaside, rivers, canals and streams which move because they all have a current.

Still Water Includes ponds, lakes and reservoirs which do not have a current.

Swimming Against a Current

It is harder to swim through moving water because a strong current can carry you the way it is moving. If you do get swept away by a strong current turn on to your back and float feet first downstream with the current. To swim across a current, get into the water higher upstream than where you want to get out, and swim diagonally.

If you need to swim through weeds, either swim slowly using Breast Stroke or scull with your hands.

SURVIVAL SKILLS

When you read about cold water (See page 13.), you will know that when you fall into very cold water, being able to swim may not be enough to save you. If you are swept out to sea, or carried away by a strong current or fall out of a boat a long way from the shore, you will have to know how to do other things to survive.

You must remember to keep calm and ask yourself these special survival questions:

- How cold is the water and how cold is the air around you?
- How strong are the winds, currents and tide? Notice which way they are moving.
- How far away from you is the shore or your boat?
- Can you swim to safety? Remember it is difficult to swim in cold water and much harder to work out how far away things are when you are in the water.
- If your boat has capsized, do you think it will stay afloat or sink? If it does stay afloat do you think you could hang on to it?
- What clothes are you wearing? Do you need to remove any?
- Can you see anything that you could use as a float; perhaps a plastic container, a ball, a piece of boat equipment, a wooden seat, a spare tyre or a rescue buoy?

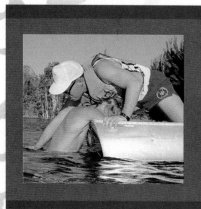

Climbing Into a Boat From the Water

The safest place to climb into a boat from the water is over the back or stern. If this is impossible then try climbing in over the side but be very careful not to capsize the boat as you do it. If there is someone in the boat already, they should try and balance the boat as they help pull you in. The easiest way to get into an inflatable boat is over the side.

REMEMBER COLD WATER CAN KILL YOU!

You need to know these survival rules.

- Make sure that your Personal Floatation Device (PFD) (See page 25.) is correctly done up.
- If you have time, enter the water calmly and carefully.
- Count how many of you there are and check who is in charge. If no one is, *you take charge.*
- Only take off any heavy clothes or boots if they make it difficult to swim.
- Try floating, sculling or treading water in as relaxed a way as you can.
- If you are wearing a PFD, lie on your back, cross your arms and go into the HELP or HUDDLE position. (See page 50.) Keep as still as you can.
- If you are not wearing a PFD, hold on to something that floats and go into the HELP position.
- Stay together.
- If you have fallen out of a boat stay with it even if it is upside down. It is much easier for a rescuer to see a boat in the water than your head!
- Use the International Distress Signal. (See page 51.)

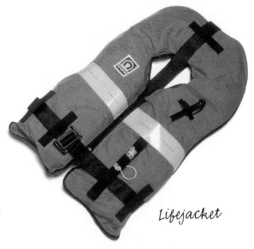

Lifejacket

Rookie Tip: Remember, you can survive in cold water if you hang on to your body heat and don't get tired.

The HELP Position

Hold something that floats against your chest with your legs straight and together. This will help you keep your body heat longer. You lose most heat from between your legs, your head and from under your arms. This position helps you keep your body heat so you can survive longer. HELP stands for Heat Escape Lessening Posture.

The HUDDLE Position

Do this when there are several of you in the water at the same time. If you huddle together you will share each other's body warmth. It will also be easier for rescuers to find you.

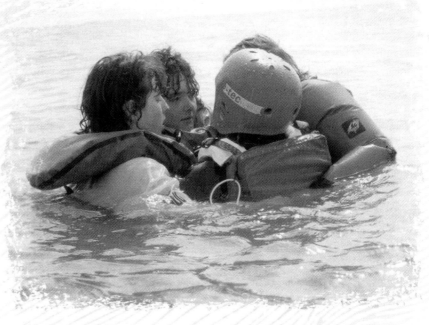

HUDDLE Position

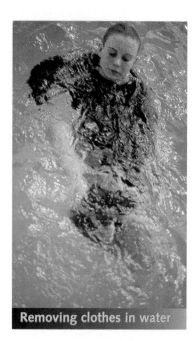
Removing clothes in water

Swimming in Clothes

If you are wearing clothes when you fall into cold water, you will find that the water trapped inside your clothes will help keep you warm if you *keep still* while you wait to be rescued. So only take off any heavy over clothes and shoes that may weigh you down in the water.

Removing Clothes

It is much harder to take clothes off when you are in the water—it is very tiring too. Be very careful if you do decide to take something off, particularly if you have to pull it over your head. Tight-fitting clothes are especially difficult to take off, so keep them on.

ICE

Never go on to frozen ponds, lakes or rivers even if you think it looks safe. If you fall through the ice, you may not be able to climb out again. If you do fall through, this is what you should do:

- Try not to panic!
- Call loudly for help.
- If the ice seems strong enough kick your legs in the water and try to slide back on to the surface.
- Lie flat on the ice and pull yourself with your arms to the bank.
- If the ice breaks and you fall in again, keep breaking it with your hands as you wade or swim to the bank.
- If you can't climb out, wait for help to reach you. Keep as still as you can and hang on to your body warmth by pressing your arms to your sides and keeping your legs together.
- As soon as you are safe, ask someone to take you to the hospital for a checkup.

*Rookie Tip: If you see someone in danger on the ice, **do not** go on to the ice to help them but go for help right away.*

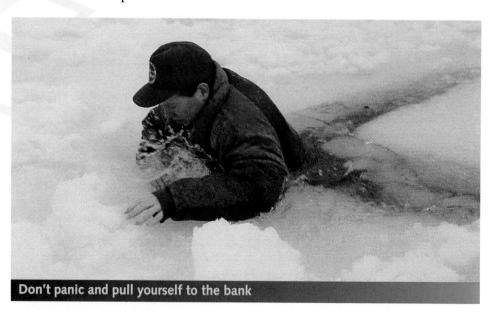
Don't panic and pull yourself to the bank

Distress Signals To Recognise

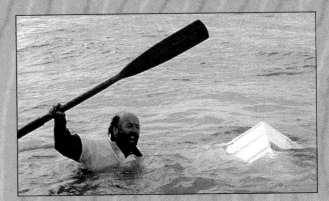

Waving an oar in the air

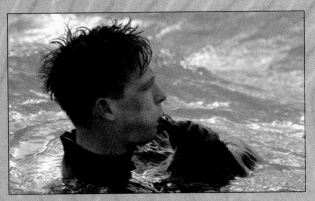

Six blasts of a whistle at one minute intervals

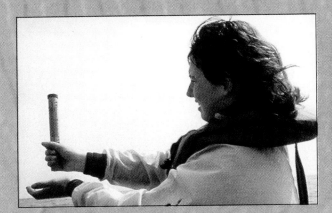

Red flares or orange smoke signals

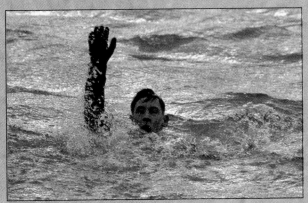

Waving one arm to and fro over your head—the International Distress Signal

PERSONAL FLOATATION DEVICE (PFD)

Always wear a special jacket called a PFD on a boat. These are usually bright red, orange or yellow so that they can be seen from a long way away. There are two types of PFD: lifejackets and buoyancy jackets. A lifejacket (See page 23.) makes sure that you float face up, but it is hard to swim in. A buoyancy jacket is more like a normal jacket and is easier to swim in. You wear it for water sports where you have to move a lot, such as canoeing or dingy sailing.

Always check that your PFD fits you, is in good condition and done up properly. Rookies should be able to tell the difference between a lifejacket and buoyancy jacket and know how to put them on and take them off.

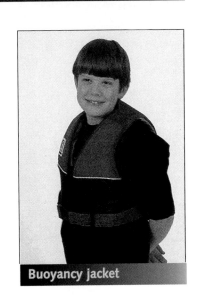

Buoyancy jacket

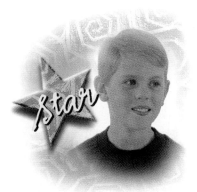

Rookie

*H*i, I'm Sam and I like the Self Rescue skills in the Rookie Programme. Doing activities where one of my friends rescues me is fun. It is also good when we practise the HELP and HUDDLE position.

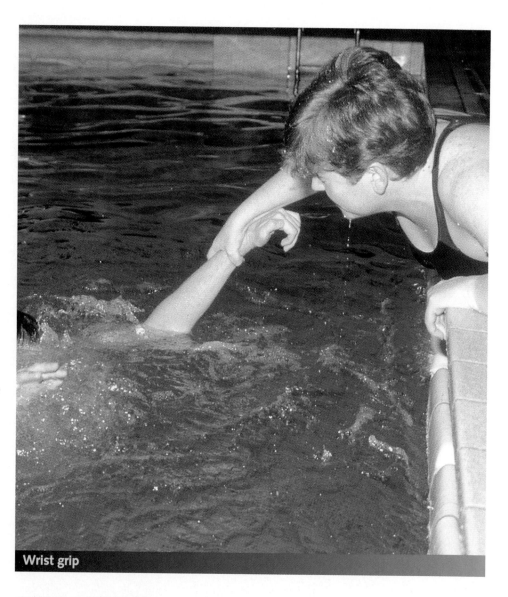

Wrist grip

BEING RESCUED

This is how you can help someone to rescue you.

- Keep calm—don't panic!
- Listen to what the rescuer tells you to do.
- Don't let your head go under the water.
- Stay afloat by moving your hands under the water and kicking your legs.
- If your rescuer reaches out her hand towards you, let her grab your wrist using a Wrist Grip.
- When you reach something that will support you, grab it firmly with both hands.
- Once you are safely on the shore, move well away from the edge.
- Know how to climb out of a pool without using the steps.
- If you have breathed in any water, go to hospital.

ESCAPING FROM A CAR UNDERWATER

If you are in a car that falls into the water try and get out through a side window before it sinks. If you can't, keep calm and help everyone in the car to:

- Unfasten any seatbelts.
- Switch on all the car lights.
- Unlock all the doors.
- Try to get up as high as you can in the car.
- When the water reaches your chin, take a deep breath and go under the water to try and open the door. Winding down the window will help.
- If you can't open the door or window, try to push the windscreen out with your feet.
- Everyone should leave the car together, linking hands as they go.
- As you float to the surface, put your head back and blow out.

Rookies should be able to describe how to escape from a sinking car.

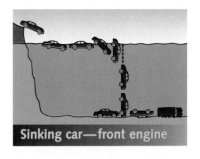

Sinking car—front engine

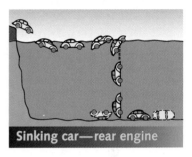

Sinking car—rear engine

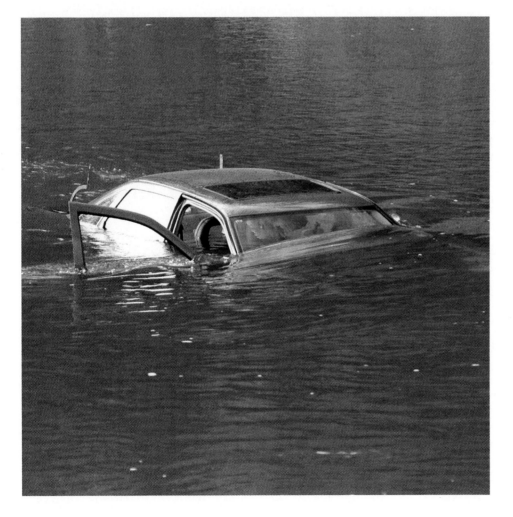

RLSS UK Rookie— Self Rescue Certificate

The Rookie Programme includes a Self Rescue Certificate for 4 Star Grades. This can be taken either on its own or as part of other Rookie training.

Now You Try It!

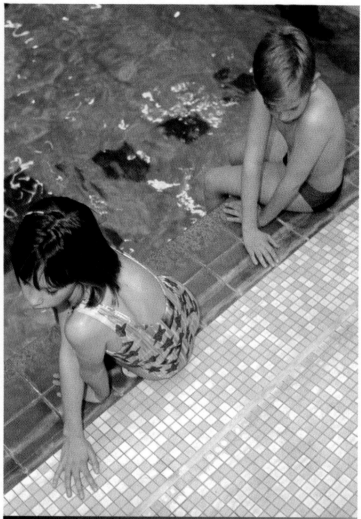

Slide-in Entry—turn towards your hands

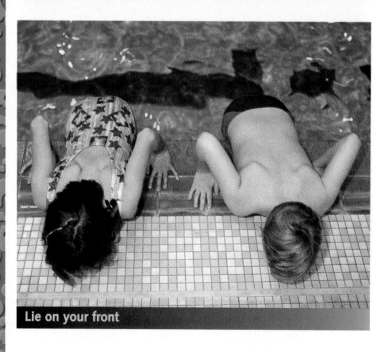

Lie on your front

Getting Into The Water Safely

Using the Steps

Face the steps and hold the rails with both hands. Go carefully, one step at a time, looking where you put your feet.

Rookie Tip: Beware of slippery steps as you climb in!

Slide-in Entry

Sit with both hands on the ground to one side of your legs. Turn towards your hands and lie on your front. Slide gently into the water.

▫ **Shallow Water**
◼ **Deep Water**

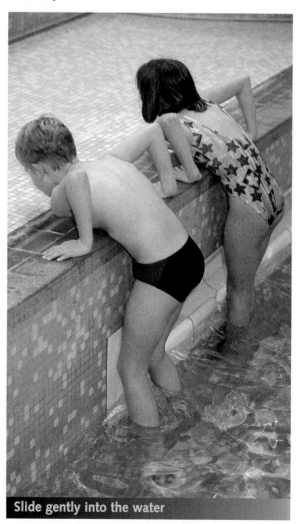

Slide gently into the water

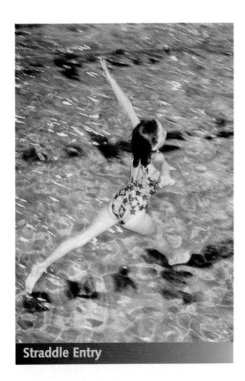
Straddle Entry

■ Straddle Entry

Put one foot forward curling your toes over the edge of the pool. Step out, lean forward and spread your arms. As you hit the water, press your arms down and scissor your legs.

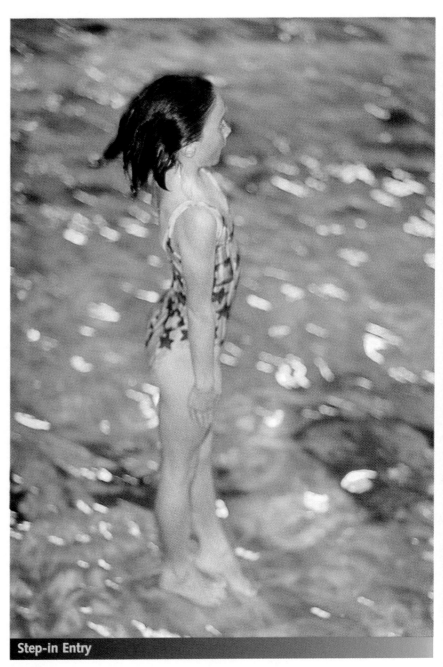
Step-in Entry

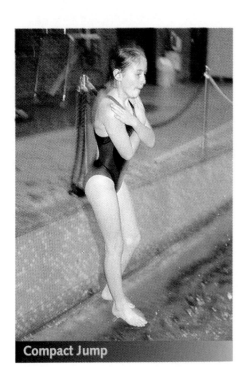
Compact Jump

■ Step-in Entry

Stand with your feet together and hands by your side. Step off the edge. Bend your knees a little as your feet touch the bottom.

■ Compact Jump

Stand with your feet together and cross your arms. Step off and point your toes. In the water, tuck up into a ball and swim to the surface.

Rookie Tip: Your head should not get wet when you are practising a Straddle Entry. Try wearing a hat and keeping it dry!

Now you try it!

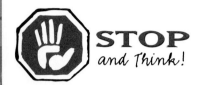

STOP *and Think!*

NEVER PRACTISE your dives in shallow water which is less than 1.5 metres deep.

Dives

■ *Sitting Dive*

Put your feet on the rail with your knees together. Press your arms next to your ears and roll forward into the water.

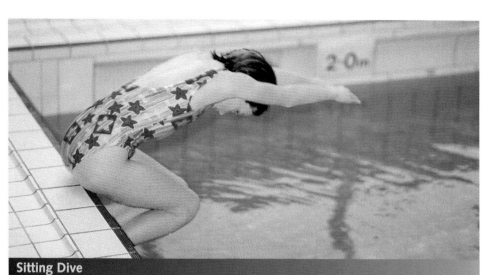

Sitting Dive

■ *Kneeling Dive*

Put one foot forward with your toes over the edge. Press your arms next to your ears and roll forward.

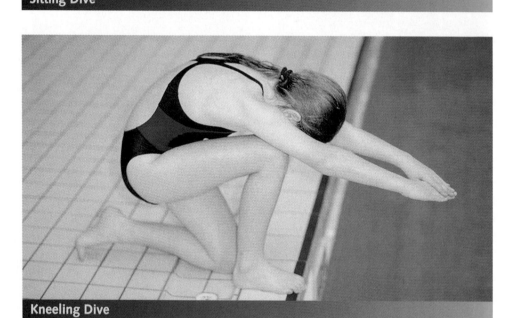

Kneeling Dive

■ *Lunge Dive*

Stand with one foot forward and both knees bent. Press your arms next to your ears and lean forward until your back foot lifts up.

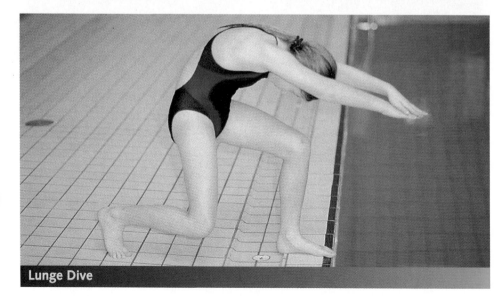

Lunge Dive

◼ *Shallow Dive*

Stand with your feet slightly apart and toes curled over the edge. Look at where you want to dive into the water. Bend your knees and swing your arms forward while pushing off with your feet. Keep your body straight, your legs together and your head between your arms.

◻ **Shallow Water**
◼ **Deep Water**

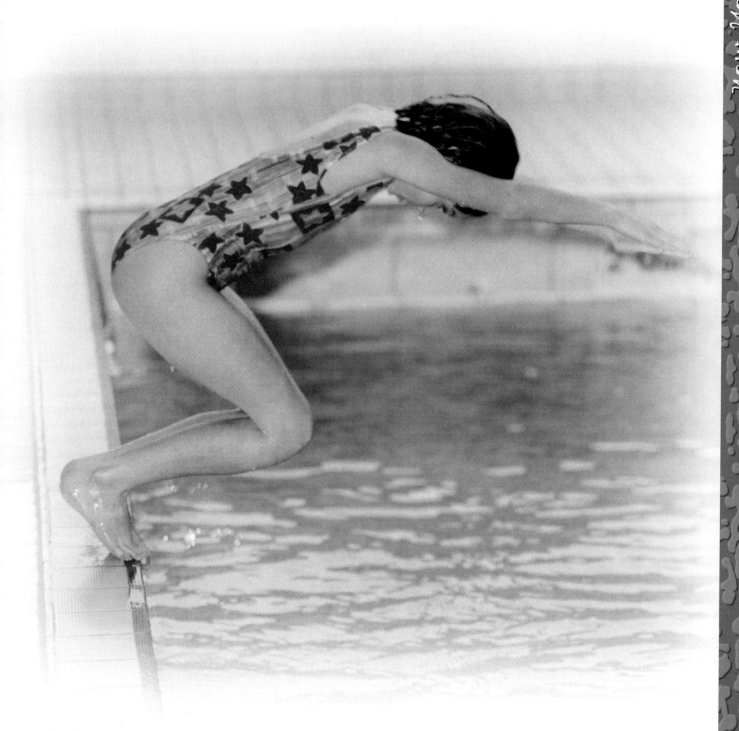

Shallow Dive

Now You Try It!

■ Falling in

Take a deep breath. Tuck up into a
ball with your chin on your chest.
Hold the top of your head with both
hands and touch your elbows with
your knees. When you hit the water,
kick your legs hard until you come
up to the surface.

☐ **Shallow Water**
■ **Deep Water**

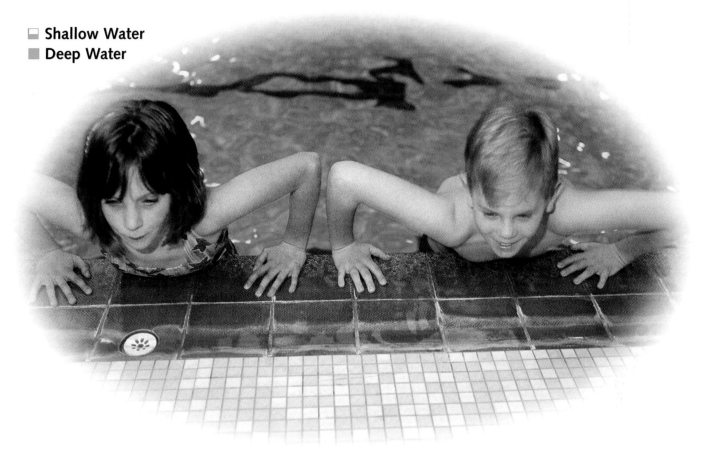

Climbing Out Without Using the Steps

☐ Put both hands flat on the poolside. Push off with your feet and push down with your arms. Lean forward, put a knee or foot on the side and climb out.

■ Put both hands flat on the poolside and let your body go under the water a little. Kick your legs hard and push down with your arms. Lean forward, put a knee or foot on the side and climb out.

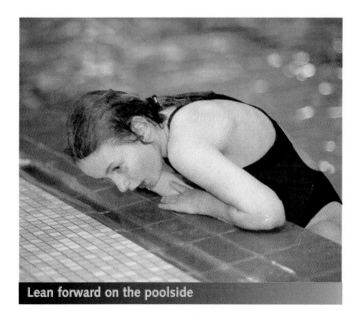

Lean forward on the poolside

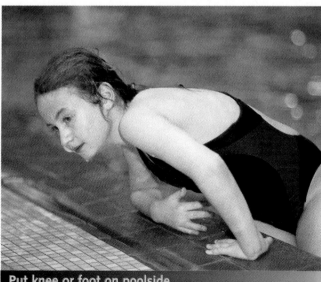

Put knee or foot on poolside

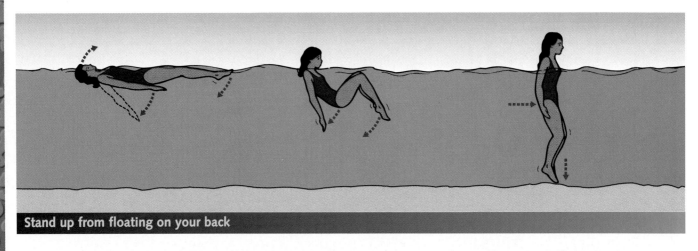

Stand up from floating on your back

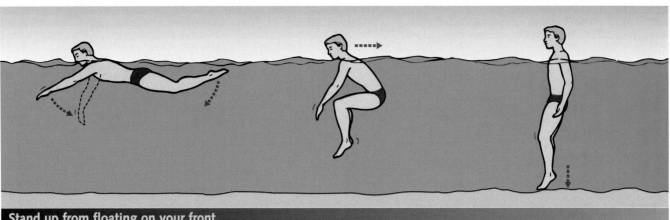

Stand up from floating on your front

Rookie Tip: It is much easier to float if your lungs are full of air, so take a deep breath before you start!

Swimming

Floating

▭ *Stand up from floating*
Float on your back. Lift your head and bring up your knees towards your chest. Press down with your hands and put your feet on the bottom. Now try it from floating on your front.

▭ *Do a Star Float*
Spread your arms and legs as wide as you can. Lie back and look up. Lift your feet off the bottom. Now try a Star Float on your front.

▭ *Float on your front and turn on to your back*
Keep your body flat in the water. Drop one shoulder and roll over.

▭ *Float in a tucked position (Mushroom Float)*
Tuck up tight like a ball.

Try this to see how well you float. Ask a friend to stand near you in shallow water. Take a deep breath and do a face down Star Float. Blow the air out of your lungs. Do you sink or float?

▭ **Shallow Water**
◼ **Deep Water**

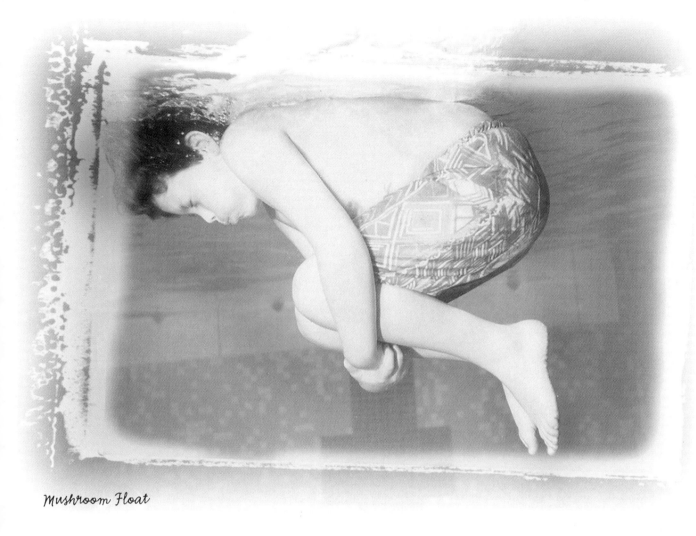

Mushroom Float

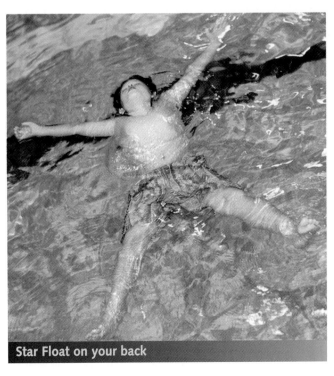

Star Float on your back

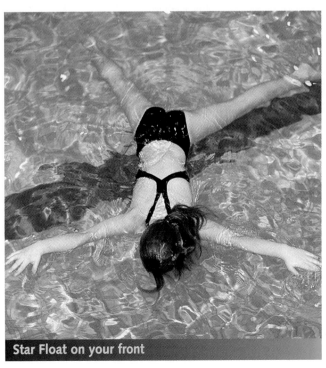

Star Float on your front

Now You Try It!

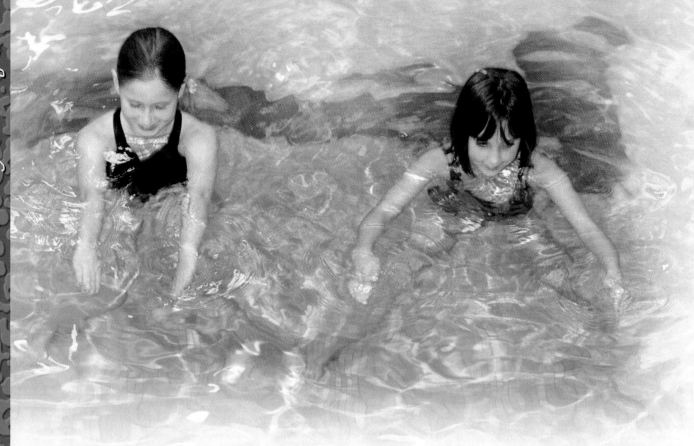

Now You Try It!

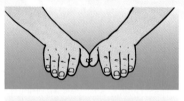
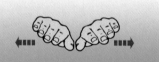
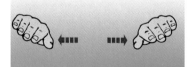
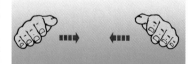
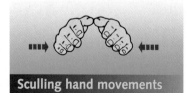

Sculling hand movements

practise your hand movements in shoulder-deep water

Sculling

Before you try this in the water, stand on the poolside and practise the hand movements.

Put your hands in front of you, palms down and thumbs touching. Tilt your hands, thumb-side down. (See the diagram.) Move them apart until they are level with your shoulders. Now tilt them the other way— thumb-side up, and move them back together. Do this a few times, slowly at first.

▣ Sculling in the pool

Practise the hand movements as you stand in shallow water.

Rookie Tip: You should feel the water push against your hands and see whirlpools around them.

Now try it in shoulder-deep water. Stretch your arms out in front, just under the surface.

Rookie Tip: You should feel your hands lift a little.

▢ *Sculling head first*

Float on your back and scull with your fingers pointing up. Keep your body flat. You can kick your legs up and down to help when you start sculling. When you can do it without kicking, put your legs together and point your toes.

▢ *Sculling feet first*

Keep your fingers pointing down.

▢ *Sculling keeping still*

Keep the palms of your hands facing the bottom of the pool.

▢ **Shallow Water**
■ **Deep Water**

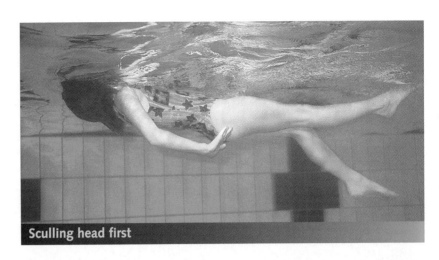
Sculling head first

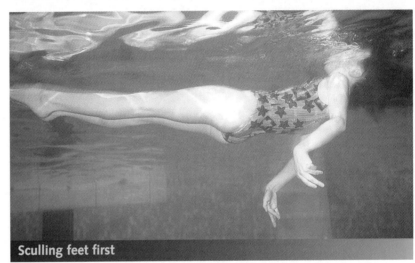
Sculling feet first

Skulling keeping still

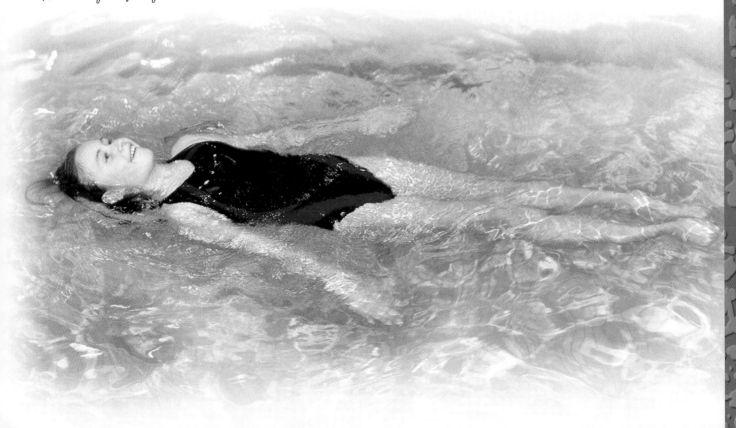

■ **Shallow Water**
■ **Deep Water**

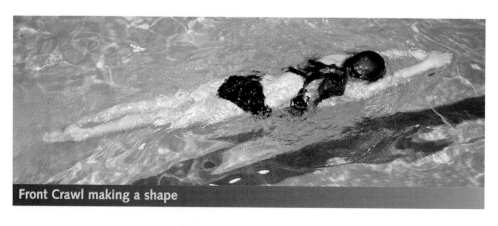

Front Crawl making a shape

Front Crawl

Rookie Tip: Stretch out like Superman.

⬒ *Make a shape*
Push off from the side with your face in the water, keeping your arms together and legs together. Point your toes and see how far you can go.

Rookie Tip: Pretend to kick off your shoes.

⬒ *Kick your legs*
Hold the rail or side with both hands, kick up and down keeping your legs straight and make your ankles floppy. Now try this holding two floats and then one float.

⬒ *Move your arms*
Stand with your chin on the water, move your arms one at a time, keeping your elbows high and your palms facing backwards under the water. Now try this walking forward.

⬒ ■ *Swim Front Crawl*
Begin by pushing off, start kicking and add your arms. Turn your head to one side to breathe in.

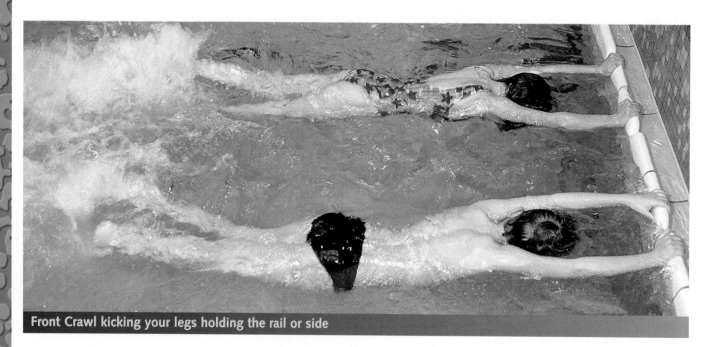

Front Crawl kicking your legs holding the rail or side

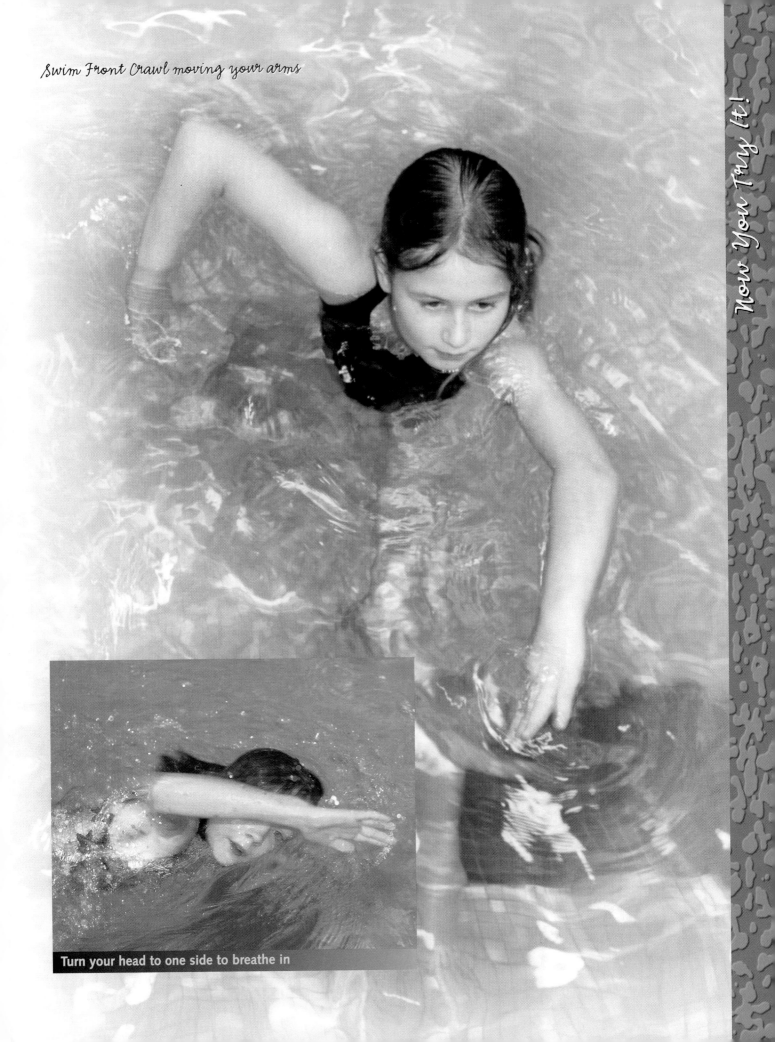

Swim Front Crawl moving your arms

Turn your head to one side to breathe in

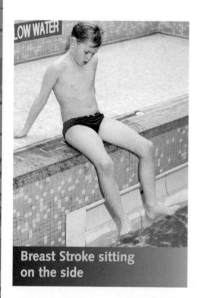

Breast Stroke sitting on the side

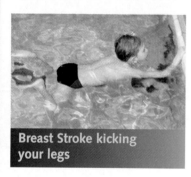

Breast Stroke kicking your legs

Breast Stroke

Make a shape

Push off the side with your face in the water, keeping your arms together and legs together. Point your toes and see how far you can go.

Kick your legs sitting on the side

Look at your feet, start with your legs straight, bring your heels towards your bottom and turn your feet out. Kick your feet round and straighten your legs.

Kick your legs

Lie on your front and holding the rail or two floats, bend both legs at the same time and kick both legs together keeping your feet turned out.

Move your arms

Stand with your chin on the water and your arms together and straight (1), pull your arms back at the same time. Keep your elbows high and your palms facing backwards under the water (2 and 3). Now try this walking forward.

■ Swim Breast Stroke

Begin by pushing off into a glide, pull your arms, take a breath, kick your legs and glide. Keep repeating this in the same order.

Rookie Tip: Keep your chin on the water.

Shallow Water
■ **Deep Water**

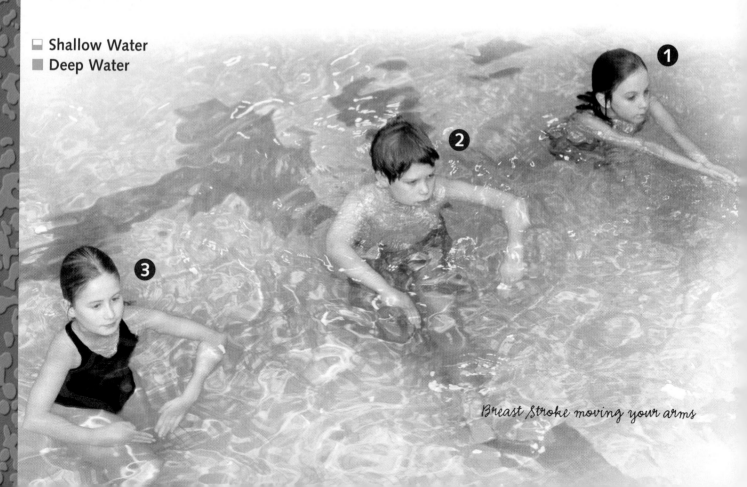

Breast Stroke moving your arms

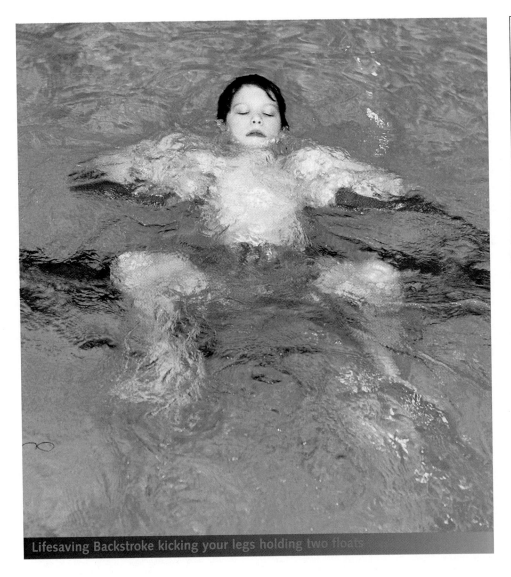

Lifesaving Backstroke kicking your legs holding two floats

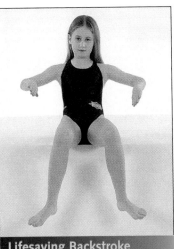

Lifesaving Backstroke kicking and sculling

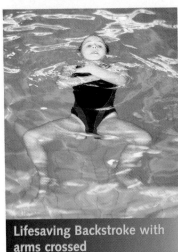

Lifesaving Backstroke with arms crossed

Now You Try It!

Lifesaving Backstroke

▢ *Make a shape*
Sit on the poolside, lean back slightly on your hands, look at your feet and turn them out as in Breast Stroke.

Kick your legs sitting on the side
Look at your feet, start with your legs straight, bring your heels towards your bottom and turn your feet out. Kick your feet round and straighten your legs.

▢ *Kick your legs*
Sit in the water holding a float under each arm. Bend both legs at the same time and kick both legs together keeping your feet turned out.

▢ ▪ *Swim Lifesaving Backstroke*
While you kick your legs, use your hands to scull. When you can do this cross your arms over your chest.

Rookie Tip: Kick your legs like a frog!

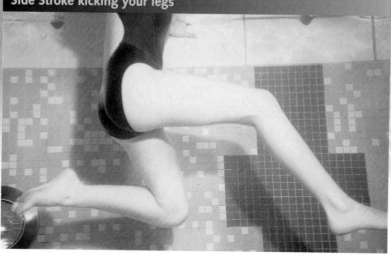

Side Stroke kicking your legs

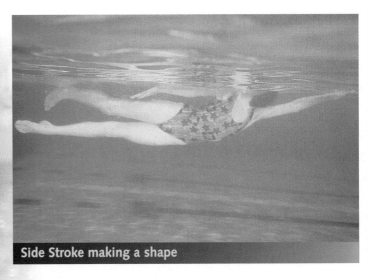
Side Stroke making a shape

Side Stroke

☐ *Make a shape*

Push off the wall lying on your side. Keep one ear in the water next to your bottom arm. Hold your top arm along your body and your bottom arm straight out.

Kick your legs standing on the side

Hold on to something, bring one knee up in front of you then push it down on the floor. Lift your other leg behind you, then push it down to the floor.

☐ *Kick your legs*

Hold the rail with one hand and a float in the other, kick both legs at the same time.

Rookie Tip: Your legs should open and close like scissors.

☐ *Move your arms*

Your top arm moves the same time as your legs open and close. Your bottom arm moves on its own.

☐ ■ *Swim Side Stroke*

Put the leg kick and the arm strokes together, remembering to stay on your side.

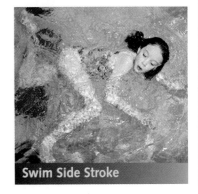
Swim Side Stroke

☐ **Shallow Water**
■ **Deep Water**

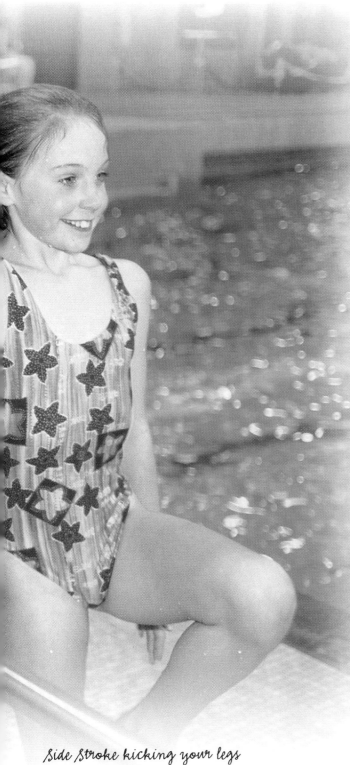
Side Stroke kicking your legs standing on the side

▢ **Shallow Water**
▮ **Deep Water**

Eggbeater Kick

Begin by sitting on the edge of the pool doing a Breast Stroke kick, moving one leg after the other. (See page 40.)

▢ Now try it in the pool. Sit in the water with your back straight and knees apart. Scull with your hands or use a float under each arm. Kick your legs one after the other in a circular pattern.

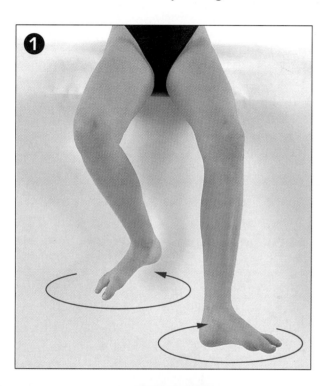

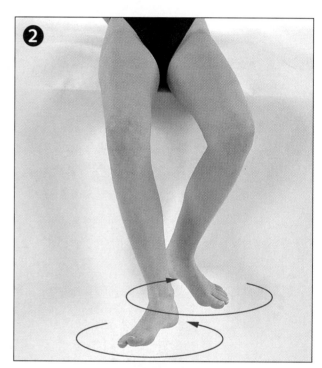

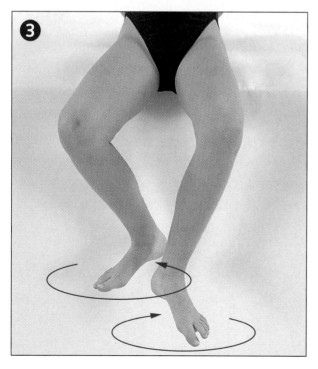

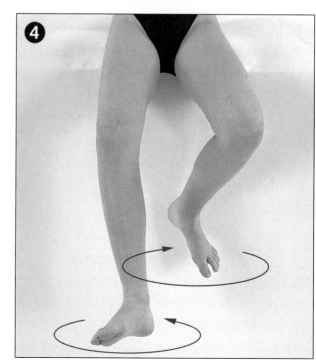

Treading Water

Make sure a grown-up is watching you with a rescue pole when you first try this.

Sit on the poolside and practise kicking your legs
You can use the Breast Stroke Kick, Scissor Kick, Eggbeater Kick or Cycling Action to tread water.

■ *Practise kicking your legs in the water*
First try this holding on to the rail with both hands. Then do it holding the rail with one hand with a float under the other arm. Now let the rail go and try with a float under each arm. Do it again with only one float and scull with your free hand.

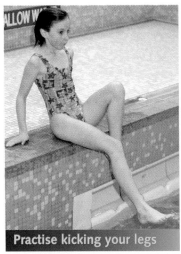
Practise kicking your legs

Rookie Tip: Cycling Action is moving your legs as if you are riding a bike.

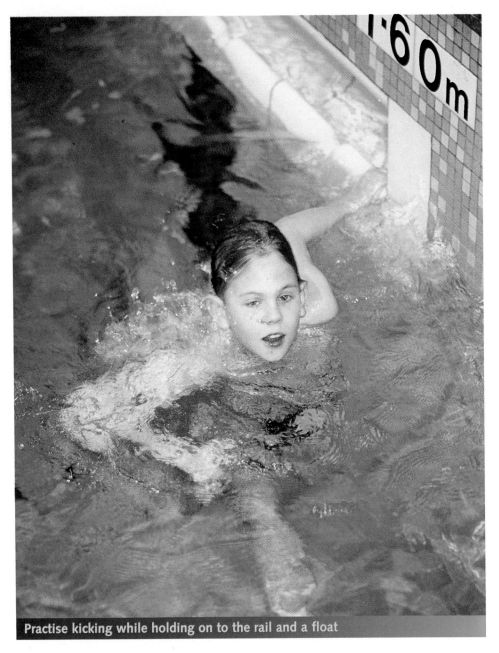
Practise kicking while holding on to the rail and a float

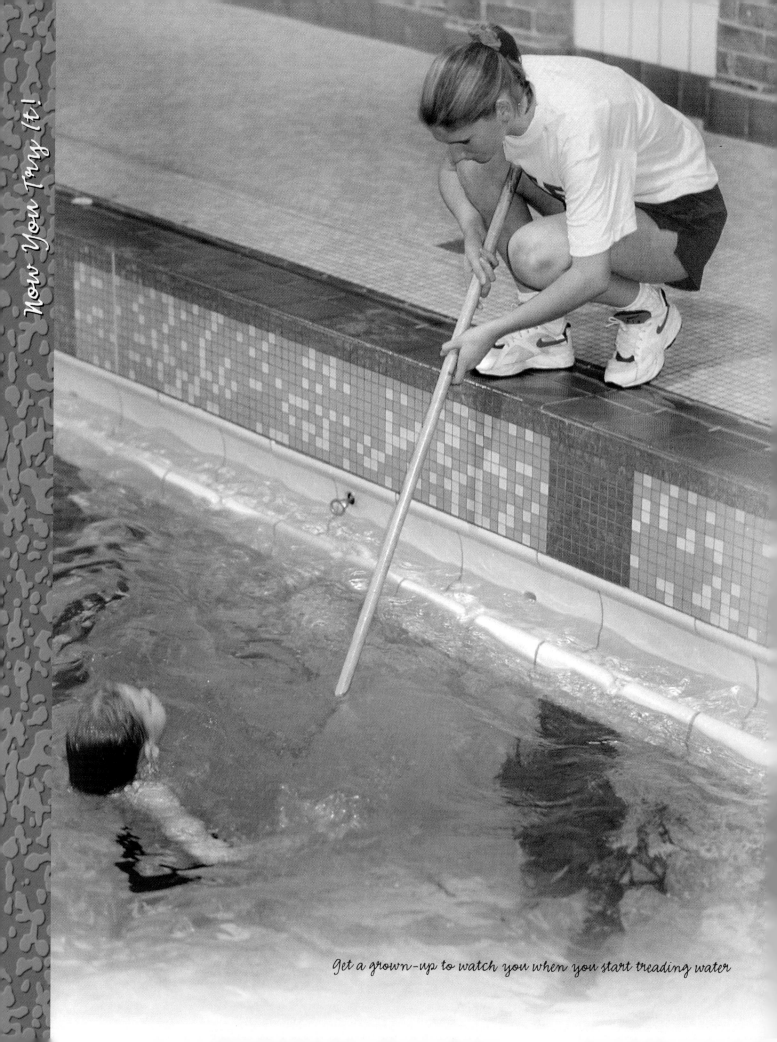

Get a grown-up to watch you when you start treading water

■ Tread water on your own

Stay close to the side and ask a grown-up to hold a rescue pole next to you when you try to do this without holding the rail or a float. Tread water and scull with both hands. Count to five and then grab the rail. Keep practising for a little longer each time.

■ Tread water without help

Try all four leg actions. Which do you like best?

■ Tread water with one hand in the air

Scull hard with one hand and use your strongest leg kick.

■ Tread water keeping your shoulders dry

Kick hard and scull hard at the same time. Now try keeping your arms dry too!

■ Tread water going round in a circle

Use your hands as paddles to move you round. Try going forwards then backwards.

■ **Shallow Water**
■ **Deep Water**

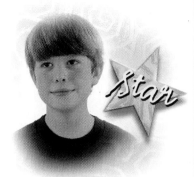

Rookie

*H*i, my name is Matthew but you can call me Matt. I have been practising treading water since I started as a Rookie and I can now tread water with one hand in the air and going round in circles. If you practice you will be able to do it as well.

Now You Try It!

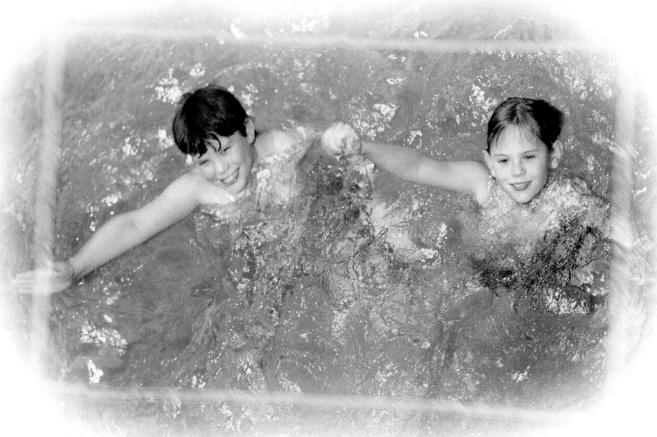

Tread water with one hand in the air

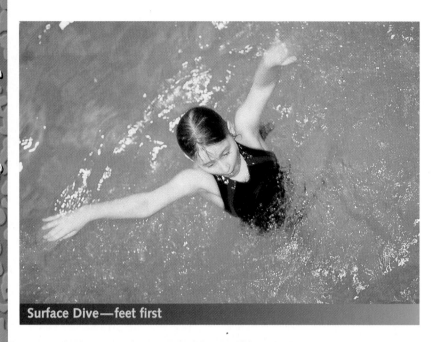

Surface Dive—feet first

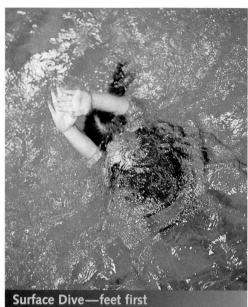

Surface Dive—feet first

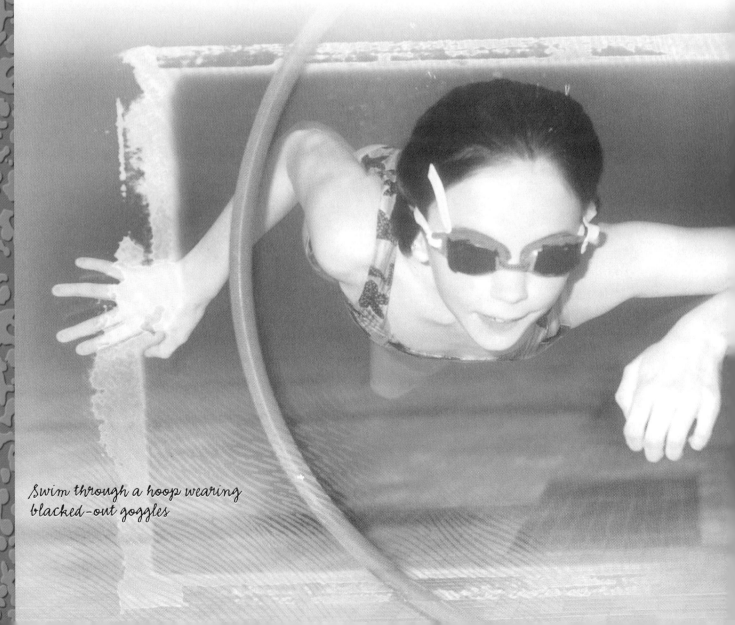

Swim through a hoop wearing blacked-out goggles

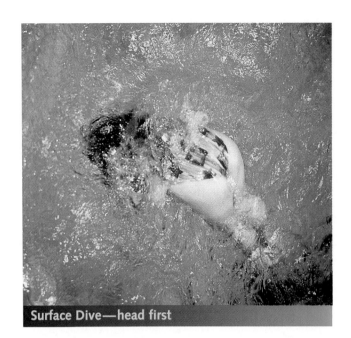

Surface Dive—head first

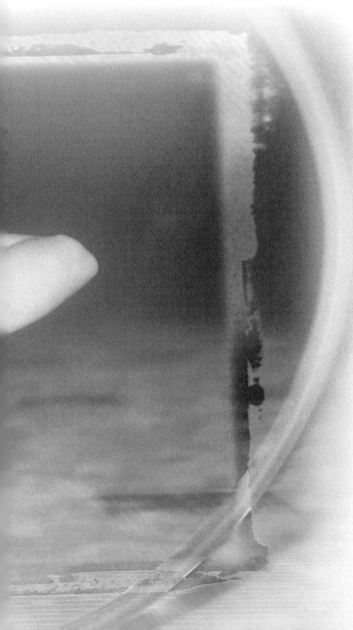

Swimming Underwater

▭ Surface Dive—Feet First

1. Start by treading water.
2. Kick hard and press down with your hands to raise your body.
3. Point your toes with your feet straight.
4. Raise your arms above your head to push your body down.
5. Take one or two small breaths just before you go under.
6. Keep your body straight and your arms above your head as you go under the water.
7. Swim underwater.

▭ Surface Dive—Head First

1. Swim to where you want to go underwater.
2. Take one or two small breaths just before you go under.
3. Put your head and shoulders under the water with your arms pushed out in front. Move your arms as if you are swimming to the bottom.
4. Bend at the waist as your head and shoulders go deeper.
5. Keep your legs straight and lift them up.

▭ Surface Dive and Pick up an Object

Clear your ears as you go down.
(See page 21.)

Rookie Tip: Never take lots of deep breaths before you dive—it is very dangerous!

▭ Swim Through a Hoop Wearing Blacked-out Goggles

Only put on the goggles when you are safely in the water. *Remember you must not try this in water that is more than 1.5 metres deep and make sure that a grown-up is in the water with you when you try this.*

Now You Try It!

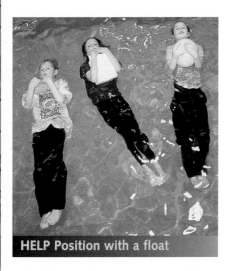

HELP Position with a float

Survival Skills

■ The HELP Position Holding a Floating Object

Float on your back holding the object to your chest. Keep your head out of the water and your legs straight together. Press your arms tight against your body.

■ The HUDDLE Position with a PFD

You need at least one other person to do this. Put your arms around each other and keep as close as possible.

▭ Tread Water Wearing Clothes

Move slowly to save energy. Try this first of all in shallow water. Make sure that a grown-up is watching you try this.

▭ **Shallow Water**
■ **Deep Water**

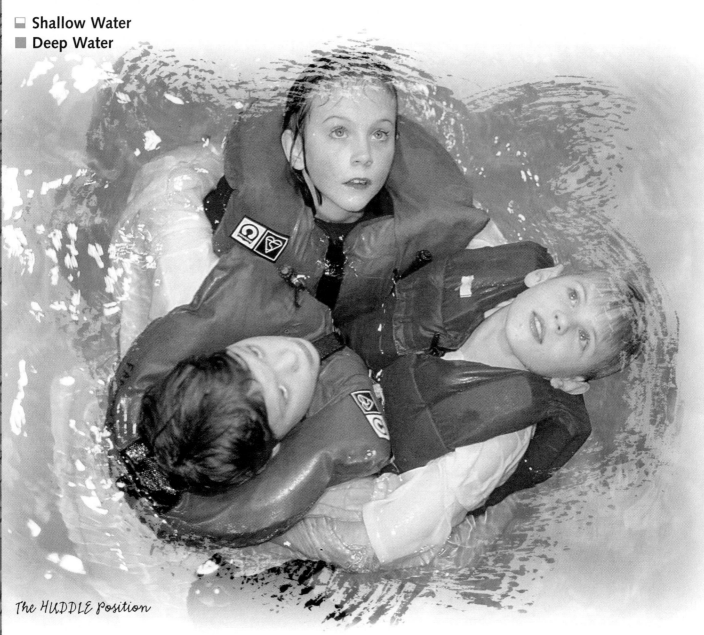

The HUDDLE Position

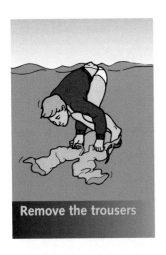

Remove the trousers

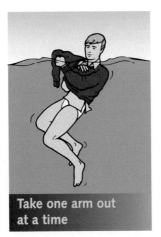

Take one arm out at a time

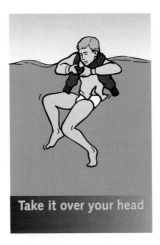

Take it over your head

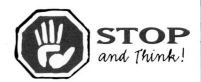

STOP
and Think!

ONLY TAKE OFF your clothes in water to practise, do not take them off in a real emergency unless they make it difficult to swim. When you practise, have a grown-up watch you.

▫ Remove Clothes in the Water

Only do this when a grown-up is watching you. Start with your shoes. Kick or push them off if you can. If you have to unfasten them, use one hand. Undo your trousers or skirt, take a deep breath, tuck up your body and pull them off. If you need to take off any clothes over your head, pull them up under your armpits, take one arm out at a time, then take them carefully over your head.

■ Fall in Wearing a PFD

Tuck up into a ball as you fall.

▫ Wade in With a Pole

Use the pole to sweep in front of you as you go into the water.

▫ ■ Practise the International Distress Signal

Wave one arm to and fro over your head. Change arms when you get tired. Try it for three minutes.

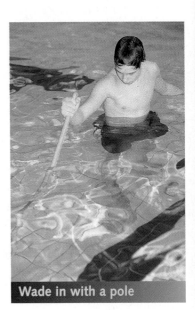

Wade in with a pole

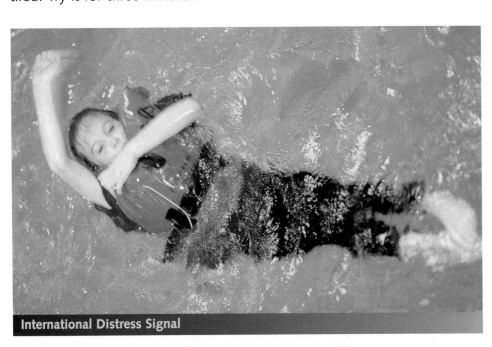

International Distress Signal

Now You Try It!

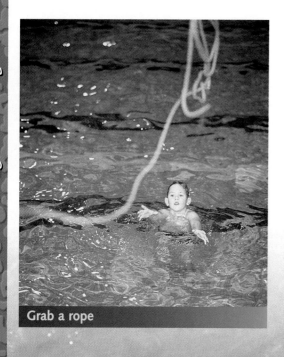

Grab a rope

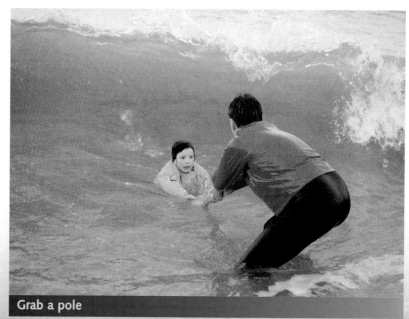

Grab a pole

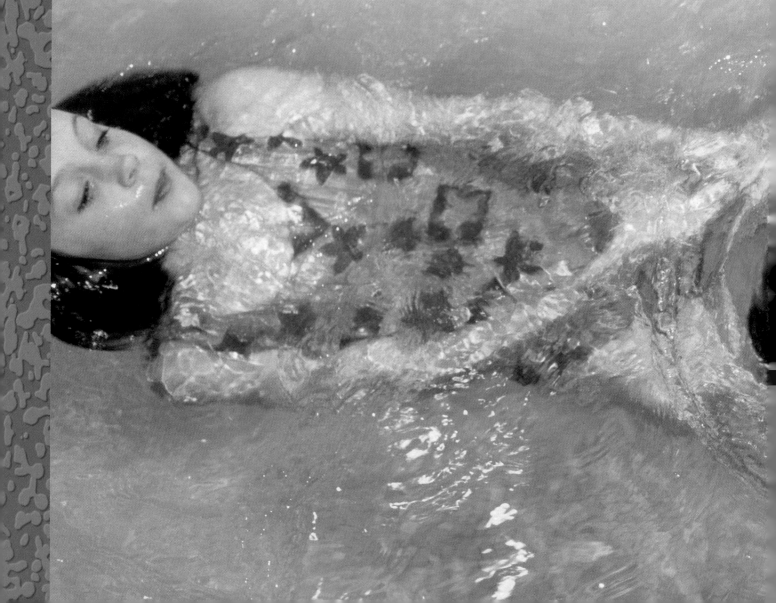

Being Rescued

■ Catch a Ball and Swim to the Poolside

Lie on your front, holding the ball under your chin with both hands. Kick your legs. Now try it lying on your back, holding the ball to your chest.

■ Grab a Rope or Line

Let yourself be pulled to the poolside, holding on with both hands. Keep your head up.

■ Grab a Pole

Kick hard as you reach for the pole. Keep your head up as you are being pulled in.

■ Practise Being Towed With a Towel or Clothing

Lie on your front holding the towel with both hands. Kick your legs. Now try it on your back, holding the towel to your chest.

practise being towed with a towel or clothing

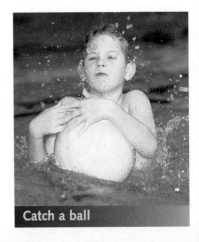

Catch a ball

Rookie Tip: Tell the lifeguard what you are doing before practising any lifesaving skills.

Now You Try It!

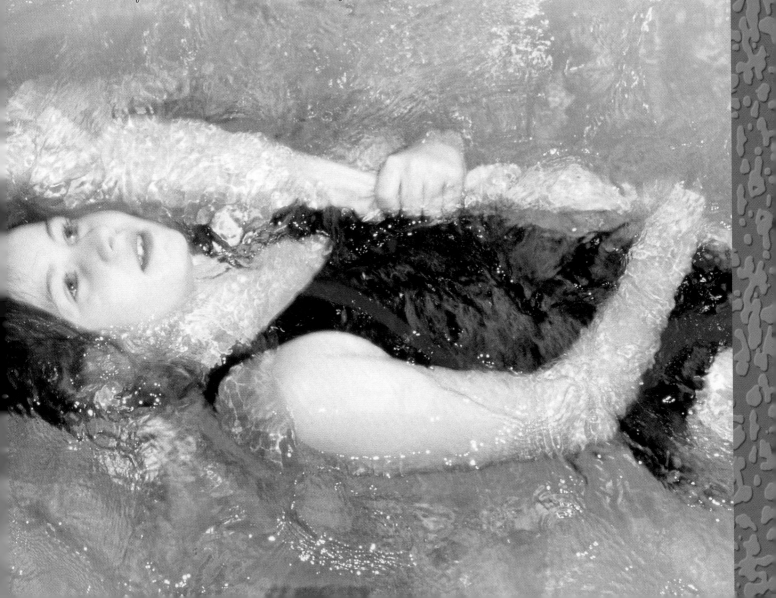

Rescue

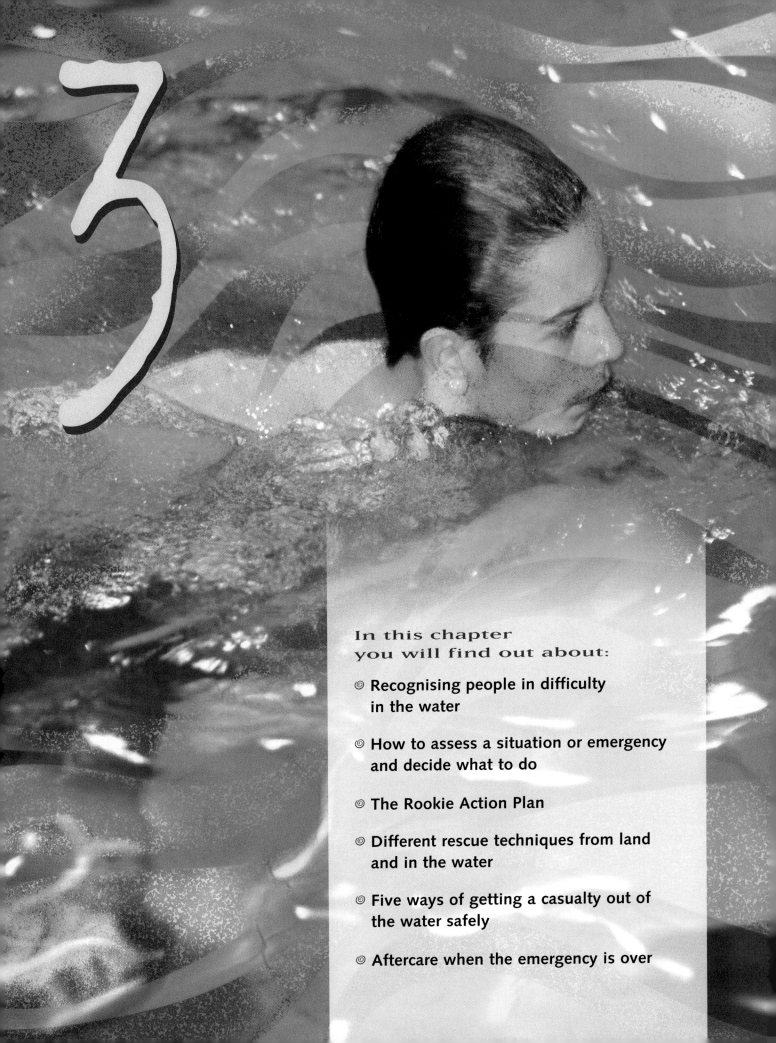

3

In this chapter
you will find out about:

◎ Recognising people in difficulty
in the water

◎ How to assess a situation or emergency
and decide what to do

◎ The Rookie Action Plan

◎ Different rescue techniques from land
and in the water

◎ Five ways of getting a casualty out of
the water safely

◎ Aftercare when the emergency is over

This chapter has two parts. The first part tells you about the skills. The second part, "Now You Try it!" shows you how to practise the skills. Have fun!

Emergencies You May See

- A person slipping on the riverbank and falling into the water.
- Someone who cannot swim very well moving out of her depth.
- A swimmer having trouble swimming back to shore.
- Someone on an airbed or inflatable drifting out to sea.

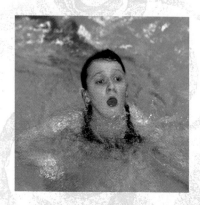

If you see someone having problems in the water, you need to know how you can help them. This chapter concentrates on one point of the Water Safety Code—Learn How to Help. You should work out a Rookie Action Plan before you rescue someone, making sure that you don't do anything which puts yourself in any danger.

There are three parts to a rescue:

1. **Assessment—**
   Before you attempt a rescue, you must think hard about what is happening so you can work out a Rookie Action Plan.

2. **Action—**
   Put your Rookie Action Plan into operation and carry out the rescue.

3. **Aftercare—**
   This is what you need to do to care for your casualty and yourself after the rescue.

Let's look at these more closely.

ASSESSMENT

If you can spot the danger before anything happens, it may mean you can rescue someone. So when you are near the water, always keep a look out for anyone who may be getting into difficulties.

Rescue Equipment Normally Used by Lifeguards

- *Torpedo buoy or rescue tube*
- *Throwing rope*
- *Throw bag*

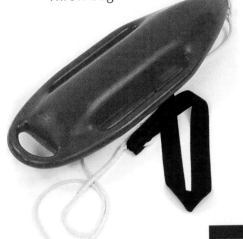

Rescue Equipment Kept Near the Water for Everyone to Use

- *Life buoy which is also called a perry buoy or a ring buoy*
- *Reaching pole*
- *Weighted throwing line*

Why Use a Rescue Aid?

- *It makes rescues safer and easier to carry out.*
- *It keeps you and the casualty afloat.*
- *It means you can reach further.*
- *It gives you something to hold between you.*

Always use a rescue aid if you have one.

Things You Can Use as a Rescue Aid in an Emergency

- *Rubber ring*
- *Plastic container*
- *Ball*
- *Tree branch*
- *Fishing rod*
- *Paddle*
- *Clothing*
- *Towel*
- *Rope*
- *Broom handle*

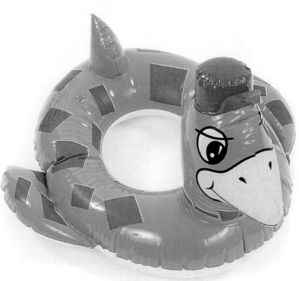
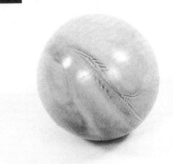
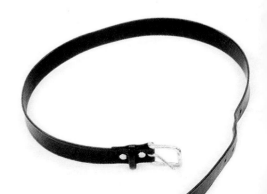

Rookie Tip: If you are not sure if you can do the rescue, fetch help. **Remember, if in doubt, leave it out!**

When you see someone who you think may be having difficulties, ask yourself these questions.

- How many people are in difficulty?
- What types of casualty are they and what problems are they having?
- What rescue equipment or rescue aids are nearby that can I use?
- Is there anyone around who can help me?
- How far away is the nearest telephone? (See page 9.)
- What have I learned to do as a lifesaver?
- How far away are the casualties?
- What is the strength and direction of the current, wind and waves?
- How deep is the water?
- If I have to, where and how can I get in and out of the water safely?

Recognising People in Difficulty

A person in difficulty in the water is called a casualty. Rookies should be able to recognise different types of casualties. There are four types and you can tell which is which by how they look and behave.

- **Non-swimmer**—a casualty who cannot swim.
- **Weak swimmer**—a casualty who is tired or who cannot swim very well.
- **Injured swimmer**—a casualty who cannot swim properly because she has been hurt.
- **Unconscious swimmer**—an unconscious casualty floating on or under the water.

Rookie Tip: Casualties can put you in danger. Non-swimmers are usually the most dangerous type of casualty because they are frightened and may well panic and grab at you.

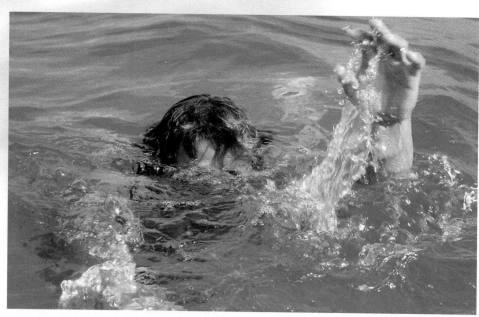

When Someone is in Difficulty

People often panic when things go wrong. If this happens, it can waste time and put other people in danger. You may be the only trained lifesaver around, so you must try and make sure that things get done properly.

The first thing to do is try to calm everyone down. Act and speak confidently, explain to them that you have received lifesaving training and that you are prepared to deal with this emergency.

Tell other people what you want them to do. Don't forget that when people have something to do they usually stop panicking. You may need to send someone to telephone for help. If you do, make sure they know what kind of help is needed and exactly where you are.

It is important that you never put yourself in any danger so make sure that you think before you do anything.

Rookie Tip: Don't try and do everything yourself— hand out jobs to other people.

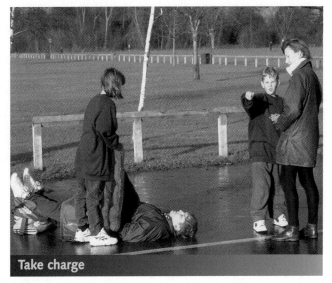

Take charge

Rookie Action Plan

Work out your Rookie Action Plan to help you decide on the safest rescue. Remember that there is always more than one way to carry out a rescue. Think of the order of the Action Plan and always do 1 before 2 etc.

If the casualty is moving with her head above the water:

❶ Shout Loudly, Clearly and Slowly

1 *"Keep your head up."*
2 *"Keep your hands in the water."*
3 *"Kick your legs."*
4 *"Look at me."*
5 *"Swim this way."*

❷ Signal

If she cannot hear what you are shouting, wave, point and signal what you want her to do.

❸ Reach

If she is close to you, do a Reach Rescue and pull her out. You can reach with a stick, clothing and lots of other things. If you are using clothing you may need to tie two items together. Make sure that you don't get pulled in yourself!

Think Before You Do Anything

Ask yourself these questions:

- *What are the dangers to me?*
- *Can I rescue her safely without going in the water myself?*
- *What is in or under the water?*
- *How big or heavy is the casualty?*
- *Am I strong enough to get her out?*
- *Can I do this rescue?*

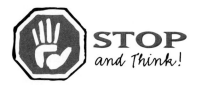

STOP and Think!

NEVER get close to a conscious casualty, only touch someone who is unconscious. Remember *ADPC*—Avoid Direct Physical Contact.

You need to be ready to defend yourself in case the casualty panics and tries to grab you. The danger is that you may get pulled under the water so be prepared to let go of the rescue aid and back off out of reach until the casualty has calmed down, and take up the *Stand-off Position*. (See page 66.)

Rookie Tip: When you are swimming, you can either hold the aid in one hand and swim one-handed, or you can tie it around your waist.

4 Throw

If the casualty is too far away to reach, use a Throw Rescue with a rope or something which floats. Make sure you stand back from the edge when you throw it. Things which float could be a ball or an empty plastic container with the lid on. Remember that a strong wind could affect the way the float is thrown.

Younger Rookies

If you are under 8 years old or if you are not a very strong swimmer do not go into the water. Go and fetch help immediately.

Older Rookies

If you are over 8 and are a strong swimmer you can continue your Rookie Action Plan with steps 5 to 8.

5 Wade

Sometimes you need to do a Wade Rescue, wading out towards the casualty. If you have to get into the water, be careful and always take a rescue aid with you. You should not wade through water that is deeper than chest level. Make sure you stay far enough away from the casualty so she can't grab you.

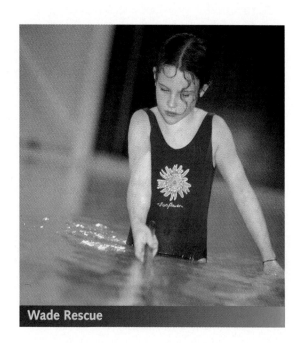

Wade Rescue

6 Row

If there is a boat nearby and you know how to handle it, do a Row Rescue. Row to the casualty and as you get close, the safest thing is to tell her to hold on to the boat while you row back to safety.

7 Swim with an Aid

If the casualty is weak, injured or too far away, use a Swim with an Aid Rescue. Swim out with a rescue aid but stay far enough away from the casualty so she can't grab you. Remember to be careful.

There are two ways to bring the casualty back to safety.

Accompanied Rescue This is where you throw the casualty a floating rescue aid, tell her to hold on to it and kick her legs. You swim alongside her, back to safety.

Non-contact Rescue Tell her to hold on to the rescue aid while you tow her to safety.

If, in either of these rescues, the casualty gets too close or tries to grab you, use the Stand-off Position.

❽ Swim and Tow

If the casualty is unconscious, you can get close to her or touch her as you carry out the rescue. (Never get close to a conscious casualty.) When you get to her, turn her over so that her face is out of the water and tow her to safety. There are three different ways to tow an unconscious casualty. You can use a Support Tow, an Extended Tow or a Clothing Tow.

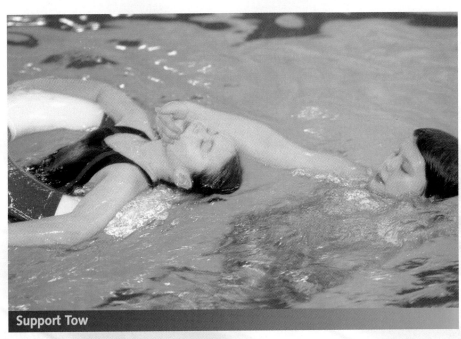
Support Tow

Remember the Rookie Action Plan
Shout and Signal, Reach, Throw, Wade, Row, Swim with an Aid, Swim and Tow!

ACTION

When you have decided on the safest rescue and have got your rescue aid, you should start to carry out your Rookie Action Plan. Be prepared to change things as you go along. Things may not happen exactly as you have planned and it is OK to change the Rookie Action Plan if you have to. For example, you may get cold, wet and tired or your casualty may fall unconscious. When something happens that you are not expecting, think whether or not your Rookie Action Plan needs changing.

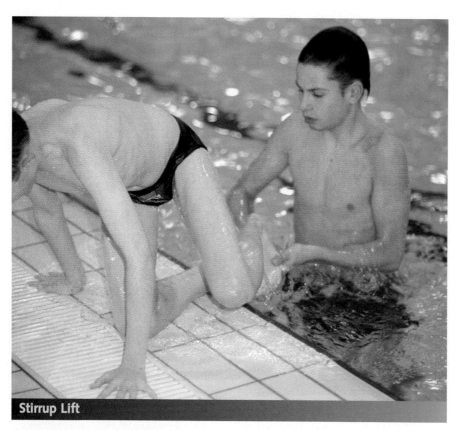

Stirrup Lift

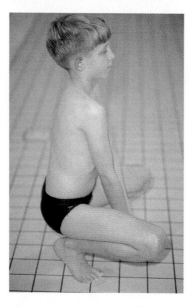

Protect Your Back

Never try to lift a casualty from the water without help. **When lifting, keep your head up, your back straight and bend your knees.** *Use the muscles in your legs, not your back.*

Getting the Casualty Out of the Water

Remember your rescue is not over until you are both safe. There are a number of ways to get your casualty out of the water and you need to pick the best one for your situation. Be careful, because this could be dangerous.

If he is conscious, use one of the following ways to get him out.

- **Tell him how to get out** This is the safest way because your casualty gets out of the water on his own. Be patient because he may be confused or in shock.

- **Assisted Walk Out** Use this in shallow water when your casualty can walk but is exhausted or in shock. Support him as he walks.

- **Stirrup Lift** Use this to get a conscious casualty out of the water where the bank is higher than the water level. Cup your hands together to make a stirrup and tell the casualty to put his foot in it. Help him to climb out, making sure that you use the correct lifting position as in the photograph.

If he is unconscious, try one of these landings.

- **Pull Ashore** Use this in shallow water when the casualty is unconscious or injured and cannot walk. Walk backwards while dragging him ashore.

When you are waiting for help at the edge put your casualty in the **Support Position.** (See page 71.) This is also a safe and secure position if you need to begin rescue breathing in the water.

Assisted Lift When you cannot get your casualty out by yourself, ask two or three other people to help you lift him out. Stay in the water while the others stay on the side. Don't forget to use the correct lifting position.

Rookies should be able to describe and demonstrate the different methods of helping a casualty from the water.

AFTERCARE

When both of you are safe, you need to give your casualty aftercare. First you need to check how she feels and then you need to give Life Support if necessary. **Life Support** is where you keep the casualty alive until other help arrives. (See Chapter 4.)

Caring for Your Casualty

- Make sure the casualty is breathing.
- Keep her warm.
- Talk to her.
- See Chapter 4, "Emergency Response," for the following:
  —Carrying out Rescue Breathing
  —Cardiopulmonary Resuscitation
  —Dealing with any bleeding
  —Dealing with shock

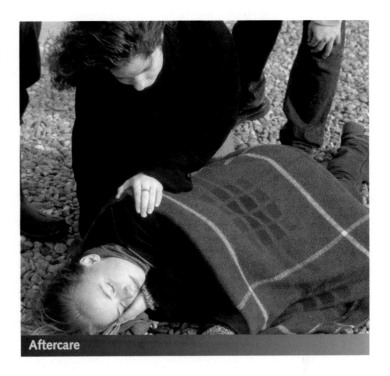

Aftercare

Remember that often the only aftercare a casualty needs is to be reassured and kept warm. If she is in shock don't give her anything to eat or drink. It is important that the casualty is checked by a doctor, even if everything seems fine.

Caring for Yourself

It is normal to feel upset afterwards because rescuing someone can be frightening. Even if you feel fine immediately afterwards you may feel upset later on. If you have trouble sleeping, feel upset or can't stop thinking about what happened, talk to a grown-up about it.

You may feel scared, guilty or angry if you were not able to rescue someone. Try not to feel guilty because you can't always rescue someone in difficulty. Remember that your own safety always comes first. Try talking to a grown-up about how you feel—it does help!

RLSS UK Rookie— Rescue Certificate

The Rookie Programme includes a Rescue Certificate for 4 Star Grades. You can take this on its own or as part of other Rookie training.

Some Very Good Reasons for Not Rescuing Someone

- *The person is too heavy.*
- *The sea is too rough.*
- *You can't remember what to do.*
- *You are not a strong enough swimmer.*
- *You don't feel ready yet.*
- *The situation seems to be too dangerous.*

Assessment

Recognising People in Difficulty

To help you recognise the four types of casualty try pretending that you are one of them—but only have a go at this if you are a good swimmer.

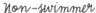
Non-swimmer

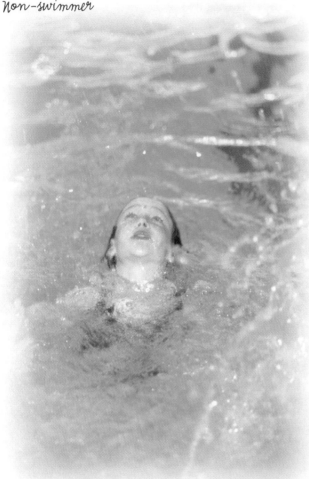

■ Non-swimmer

Reach up with your hands above your head and at the same time try to touch the bottom with your feet. Don't use your arms or legs for support. Open your eyes wide and try to look scared. Don't help the rescuer.

■ Unconscious swimmer

Take a deep breath and float face down with your eyes closed.

■ Weak swimmer

Act as if you are very tired and only swim doggy paddle. Use your arms and legs for support but let your head go under the water from time to time. Wave and call for help.

■ Injured swimmer

As you swim hold on to your injured leg. Act and call out as if you are in pain. Now try it again, but this time hold an injured arm, shoulder or head.

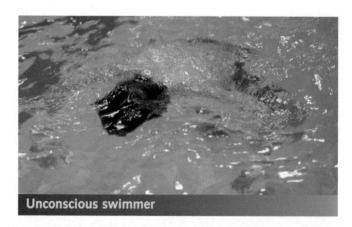
Unconscious swimmer

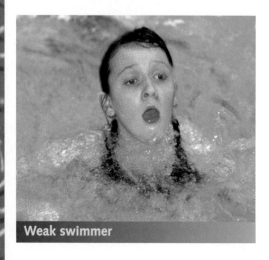
Weak swimmer

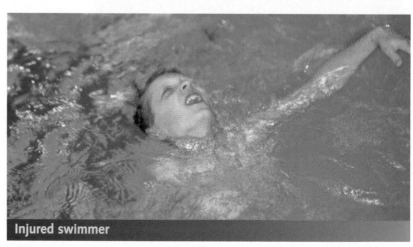
Injured swimmer

Rookie Action Plan

Rescues From the Poolside

■ *Reach Rescue*
Lie down and hold on to something firm or ask someone to hold your legs. Reach out to your partner using a pole, piece of clothing or your hand. Pull her to safety.
Try all three.

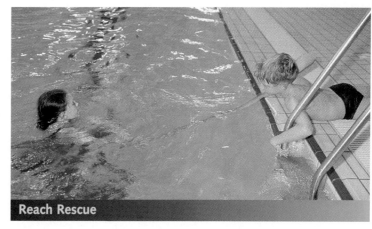
Reach Rescue

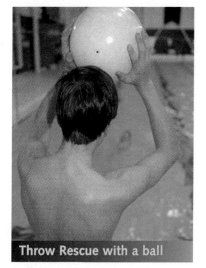
Throw Rescue with a ball

■ *Throw Rescue with a ball, container or life buoy*
Stand back from the edge and aim at a spot in front of your partner. Throw overarm or underarm, whichever you do best. Tell your partner to grab the aid and kick her legs.

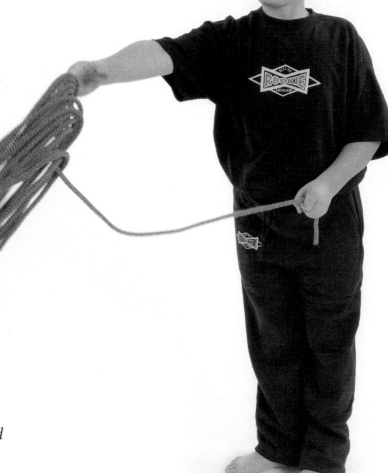

■ *Throw Rescue with a rope*
Stand back from the edge of the pool and coil the rope. Hold on to one end and throw the coiled rope over the head of your partner. Tell her to hold on and kick her legs. Pull her in and then either tell her how to get out of the water or help her out.

☐ **Shallow Water**
■ **Deep Water**

Rookie Tip: When you throw a rescue aid be very careful not to hit your partner.

Now You Try It!

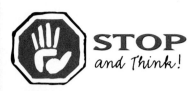

STOP *and Think!*

THESE ARE ONLY for strong swimmers over 8 years old.

Rescues in the Water

Wade Rescue using a pole

Get in slowly, using the pole in front of you as you wade. When you are close to your partner, reach towards her with the pole keeping it away from her face. Stay away from your partner until you have returned to safety.

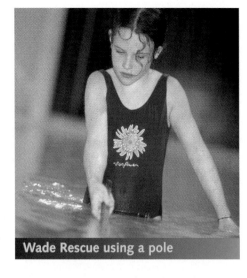

Wade Rescue using a pole

Back off when your partner tries to grab you

Ask your partner to grab at you as you swim towards him. As he does so, you should throw your head back and swim backwards kicking hard. Stay out of his reach.

Stand-off Position

Swim towards your partner and stop at least four arm lengths away. Scull with your hands and put one leg forward, slightly bent.

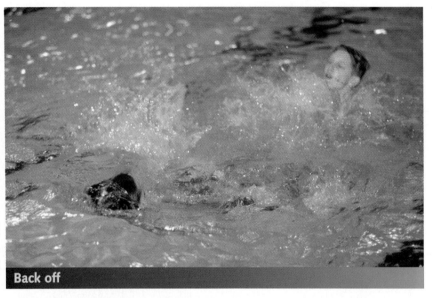

Back off

Stand-off Position

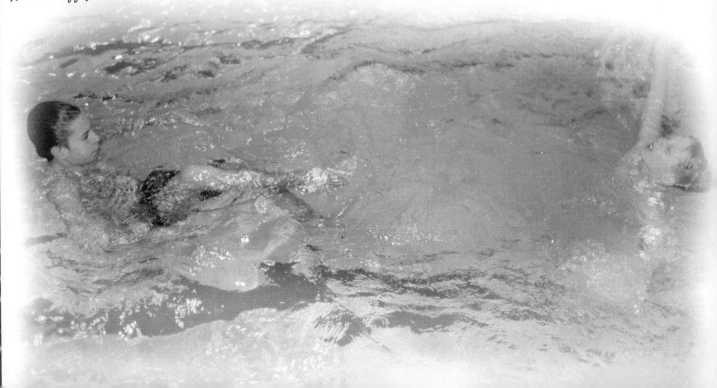

■ *Swim with an Aid Rescue (accompanied)*

Get into the water carefully and swim holding a ball or container. Do not get any nearer than four arm lengths and go into the Stand-off Position. Float or throw the aid in front of your partner. Tell him to hold it against his chest and kick his legs. Keep talking to him as you swim with him to safety but keep out of reach. At the side, help him out or tell him how to get out on his own.

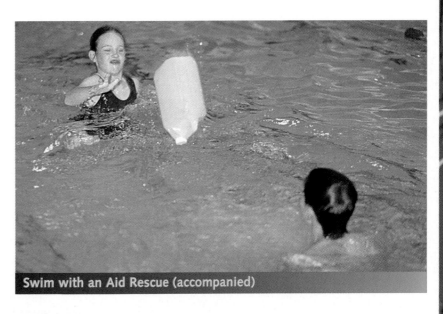

Swim with an Aid Rescue (accompanied)

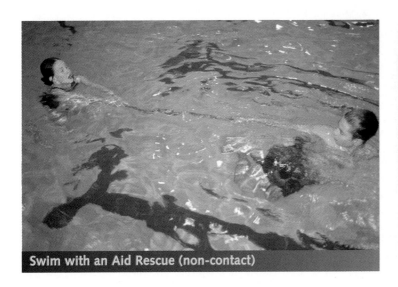

Swim with an Aid Rescue (accompanied)

■ *Swim with an Aid Rescue (non-contact)*

Enter the water carefully and swim holding a piece of clothing or a pole. Go into the Stand-off Position in front of your partner. Give one end of the aid to your partner and tell her to hold on to it and kick her legs. Tow your partner to safety using Side Stroke or Lifesaving Backstroke. Keep the arm you are towing with straight. When you reach the side help her out or tell her how to get out.

▢ **Shallow Water**
■ **Deep Water**

Swim with an Aid Rescue (non-contact)

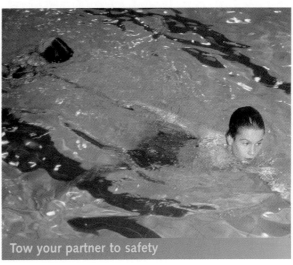

Tow your partner to safety

Now You Try It!

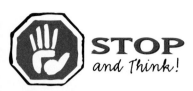

DO NOT USE these rescue methods on a conscious casualty. When you are practising ask your partner to pretend to be unconscious.

🔲 **Shallow Water**
⬛ **Deep Water**

Swim and Tow

🔲 ⬛ *Turn an unconscious casualty*

Stand or tread water on one side of your partner. Roll him over by his shoulders. Support his head and chin as you get ready to tow him.

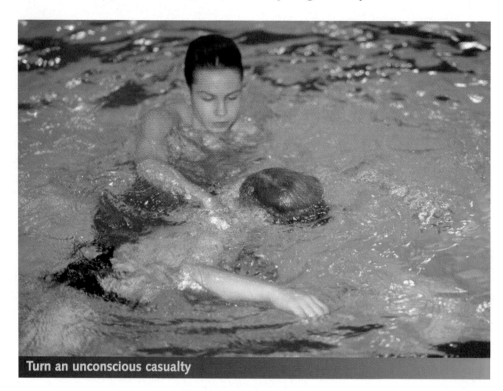

Turn an unconscious casualty

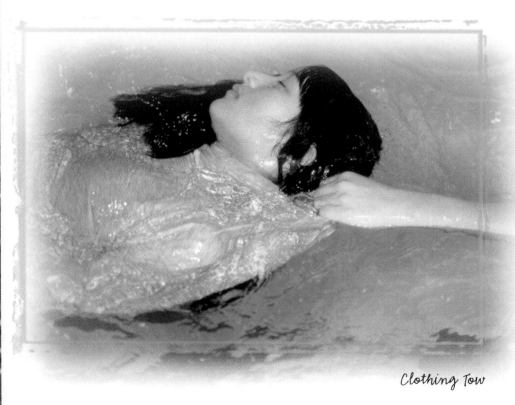

🔲 ⬛ *Clothing Tow*

Your partner will need to wear a shirt for this. Stand or tread water behind your partner and loosen any tight clothing around her neck. Grab a handful of fabric behind her neck and tow using Side Stroke or Lifesaving Backstroke. Relax your towing arm, with your partner right behind you.

Clothing Tow

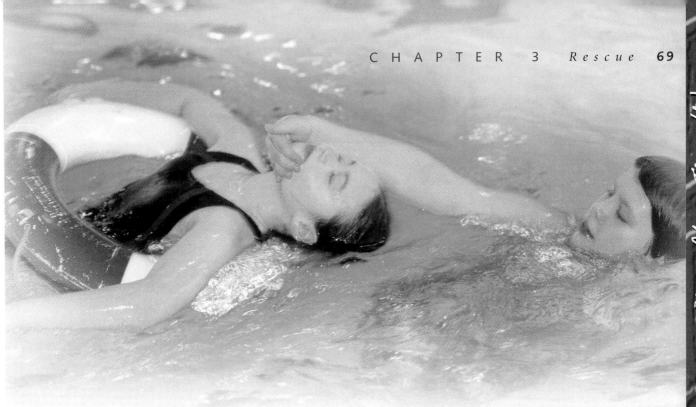

Support Tow

❑ ■ Support Tow

Stand or tread water behind your partner and put a life buoy under her shoulders. Cup one hand around her chin, keeping your hand clear of her throat. Tow her to safety using Side Stroke or Lifesaving Backstroke.

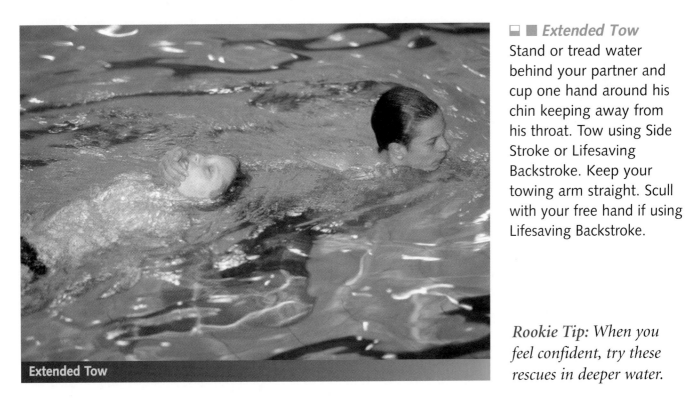

Extended Tow

❑ ■ Extended Tow

Stand or tread water behind your partner and cup one hand around his chin keeping away from his throat. Tow using Side Stroke or Lifesaving Backstroke. Keep your towing arm straight. Scull with your free hand if using Lifesaving Backstroke.

Rookie Tip: When you feel confident, try these rescues in deeper water.

Now You Try It!

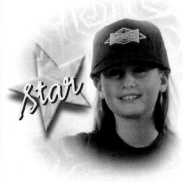

Rookie

*H*i, my name is Alice and I have been a Rookie for a couple of years. I like practising the rescues, and one of my favourites is the Pull Ashore. When you try it just be completely relaxed and let your partner pull you to safety.

Action

Getting the Casualty Out of the Water

Tell her how to get out

Say: *"Hold on with two hands when you get to the side. Put your hands on the poolside with your palms down. Push down with your hands, kick your legs and move your head forward. Get clear of the water and sit down facing away from the edge."*

▫ Assisted Walk Out

Slide your head under your partner's armpit and hold her arm over your shoulder. Put your other hand around her waist. Walk ashore supporting her.

▫ Pull Ashore

Float your partner up the beach until the water reaches your waist. Lean your partner's back against your front. Put your arms under her armpits and hold her wrists on her chest keeping your back straight. Now walk backwards, dragging your partner. Lower her gently to the ground in a safe position away from the water.

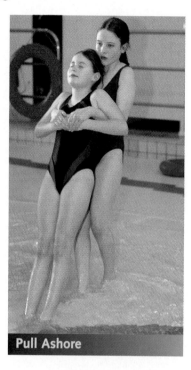

Pull Ashore

▫ Stirrup Lift

Support your partner against the edge of the pool and move to one side of him. Reach down and cup one hand under his foot or knee. Tell him to put his hands palm down on the side. Keep your head up, your back straight and bend your knees. On the count of three, lift with your hands while your partner pushes down with his hands and leans forward to climb out.

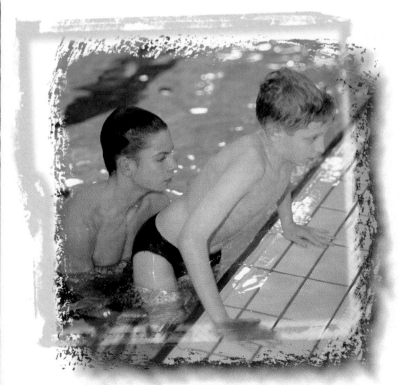

Stirrup Lift

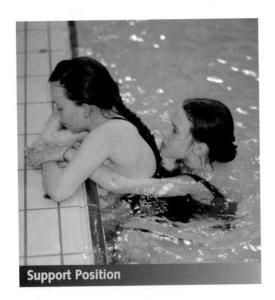

Support Position

❑ ◼ *Support Position*

Rest your partner's head against your shoulder. Put your arms under her armpits and grip the poolside with both hands with your partner facing the side. Give extra support by putting your foot on the wall and letting her sit on your knee.

❑ ◼ *Assisted Lift*

Hold your partner in the Support Position and call for help. Ask your two helpers to stand on the side and hold your partner's wrists and elbows. On your command, everyone lifts at the same time until your partner's thighs are level with the top of the side. Bend your partner at the waist and lower her body to the ground, making sure you support both her head and her body. Lift your partner's legs on to the side and move her away from the side by turning her body and legs. If you have three helpers, get one of them to support your partner's head when you lift.

Rookie Tip: When you feel confident, try these rescues in deeper water.

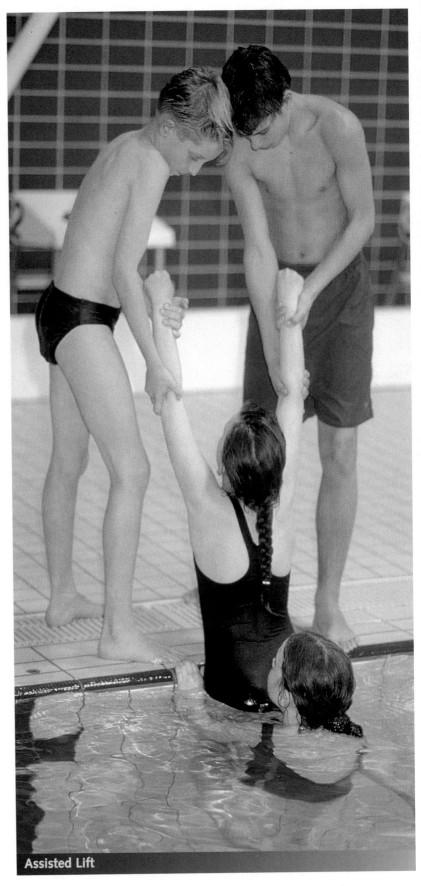

Assisted Lift

Now You Try It!

Emergency Response

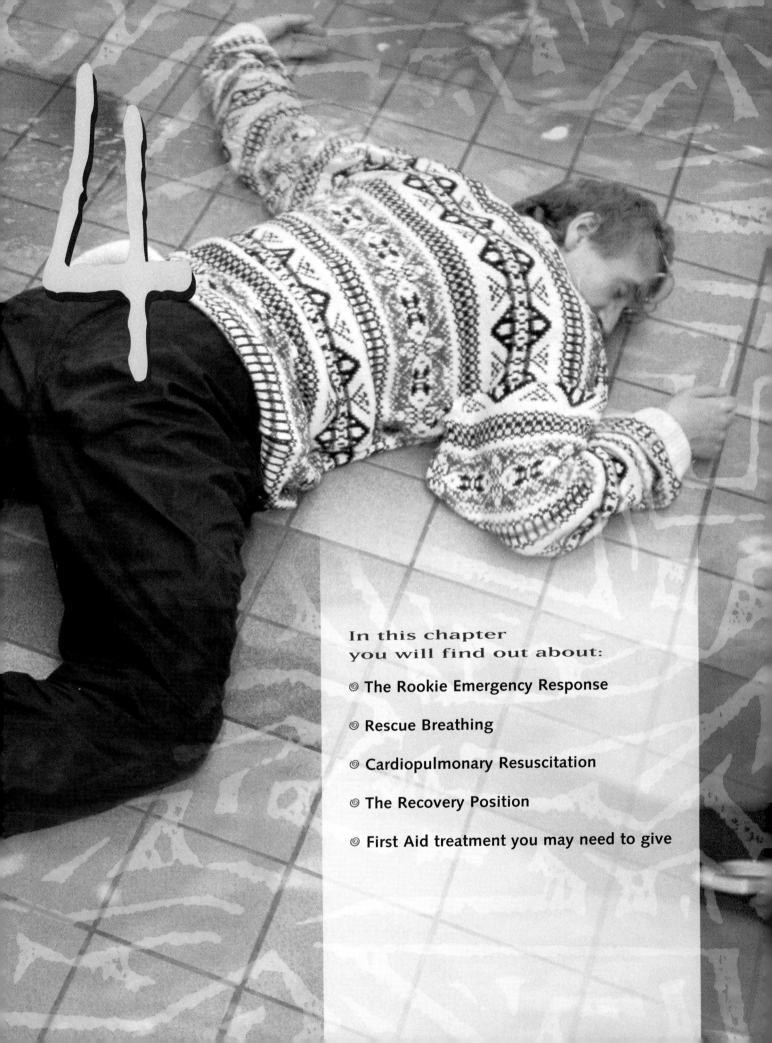

4

**In this chapter
you will find out about:**

◎ **The Rookie Emergency Response**

◎ **Rescue Breathing**

◎ **Cardiopulmonary Resuscitation**

◎ **The Recovery Position**

◎ **First Aid treatment you may need to give**

Rookie Tip: You may not have much time, so it is important you know what to do!

Emergencies do happen and you need to be ready for them. Practise the Rookie Emergency Response so you know how to deal with them. This way you can help save lives. This Chapter shows you how to respond to an emergency.

Emergency Response is the help you can give your casualty before the Emergency Services arrive. There are two types of Emergency Response:

❶ **Life Support** where you keep the casualty alive.

❷ **First Aid** where you treat the casualty's injuries.

Hygiene

Hygiene is very important. When you are dealing with an injured casualty you should wash your hands thoroughly with soap or, if you can, wear disposable gloves. Although it is quite safe to carry out Rescue Breathing and CPR, try not to get any of the casualty's blood on your skin.

Emergency Response

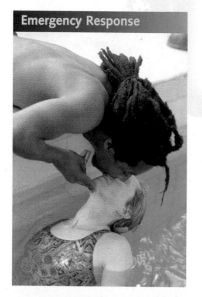

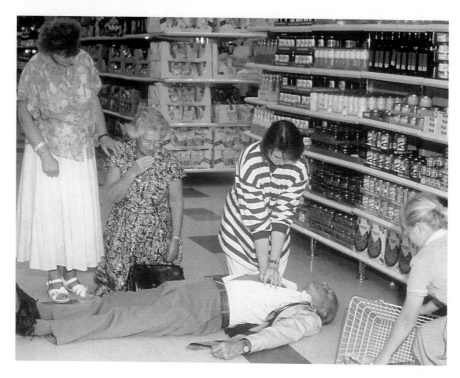

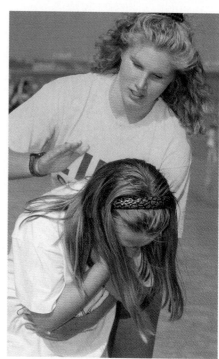

Rookie Emergency Response

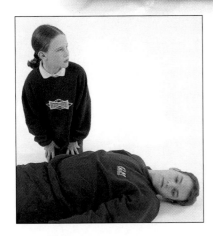

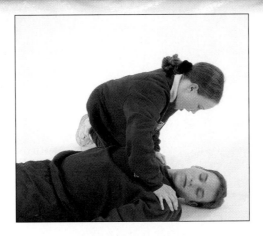

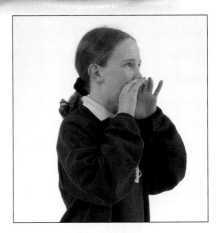

1. **Check for Danger.**
   Look around carefully and ask yourself if you should continue or move with your casualty to a safer place.

2. **Check for Response.**
   Ask loudly. "*Are you all right?*" and shake his shoulders gently. If he answers or moves, check to see if he has any other injuries and leave him where he is. Keep an eye on him and get help if necessary.

3. **Shout for help.**
   If the casualty does not respond or move, you need to shout for help as loudly as you can, until someone comes.

Now follow the ABC of Rescue Breathing and CPR.

4. **Check if his Airway is open so he can breathe easily.**
   Undo any tight clothing around his neck and check to see if he has anything in his mouth. If he has, take it out. Place two fingers under the end of his chin and the other hand on his forehead. Lift his chin and tilt his head back so that his tongue is not blocking his airway.

5. **Check if he is Breathing.**
   Place your cheek close to the casualty's mouth for five seconds. Can you see his chest moving? Can you hear him breathing? Can you feel his breath on your cheek?

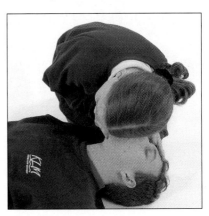

Rookie Tip: To help you remember these first very important five points, think of DR ABC: (Danger, Response, Airway, Breathing, Circulation).

If he is breathing but unconscious, put him into the Recovery Position (See page 80.) and dial 999 for the Emergency Services. When you return, keep watching him until the Emergency Services arrive and from time to time check his breathing. Gently reassure him.

If he is not breathing

6. **Check his blood Circulation by feeling his pulse.** A pulse is where you can feel the blood being pumped around his body by his heart. To check if his heart is beating you should:
   - Place two fingers in the middle of the front of his neck.
   - Slide them down to your side of his neck until you feel a large muscle.
   - Press down gently to feel for a pulse.
   - Feel for five seconds.

7. **If you can feel his pulse but he is not breathing, you should begin Rescue Breathing.** This is when you blow air into your casualty's mouth or nose to pump up his lungs. Remember, you only do this if he has stopped breathing.
   - Make sure his head is tilted back (1).
   - Pinch closed the nostrils on each side of his nose (2).
   - Take a big breath and place your mouth right over his mouth leaving no gaps (3).
   - Blow slowly for about two seconds until you see his chest rise.
   - Take your mouth away and let him breathe out on his own. *Then repeat.*

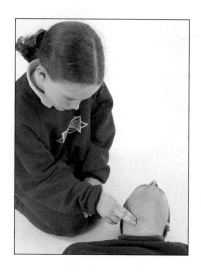

An unconscious person is someone whose brain is not thinking and whose body cannot move.

Do this 10 times, then dial 999 for the Emergency Services. Come straight back and check the casualty's breathing and pulse again. If he is still not breathing but you can feel a pulse you should continue Rescue Breathing.

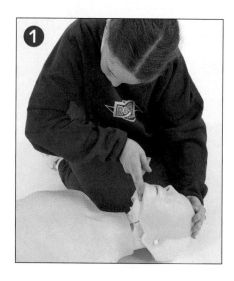

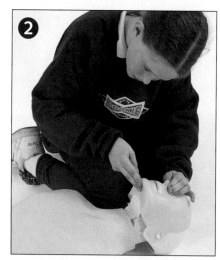

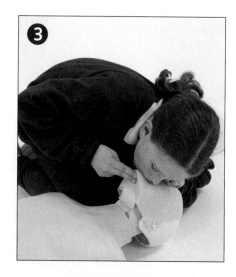

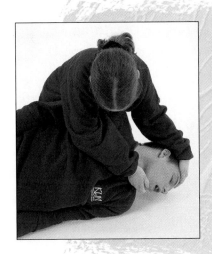

If the casualty is sick, don't worry.

- Roll him away from you, turning his face to the ground and keeping hold of his shoulder while the sick comes out of his mouth.
- Clean out any sick left in his mouth with your fingers, making sure that it is completely clear.
- Turn him on to his back again and continue Rescue Breathing.

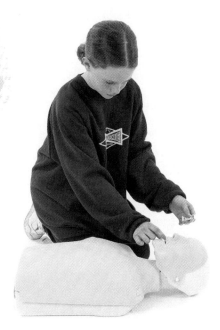

8. **If you cannot feel a pulse, dial 999 for the Emergency Services,** then come back and give 2 breaths of Rescue Breathing and begin Cardiopulmonary Resuscitation (CPR). CPR combines Rescue Breathing with pressing on the casualty's chest to make the heart keep pumping the blood around his body.

   - Place two fingers just above the bottom of his chest bone (1).
   - Slide your other hand down the chest bone to your two fingers. Do not split your fingers (2).
   - Lock your fingers together and lock your elbows together, keeping your arms straight.
   - Lean forward and press firmly down 15 times, about 4 to 5 centimetres each time (3).
   - When you press, count "one *and* two *and* three *and* four" up to 15, a bit faster than once every second.

Practise Rescue Breathing and CPR on a special resuscitation manikin. Make sure it is cleaned, as recommended by the manufacturer, before you begin. Do not practise on a person.

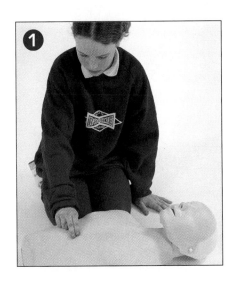

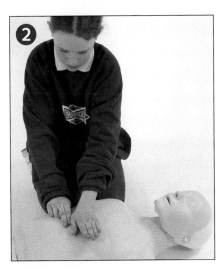

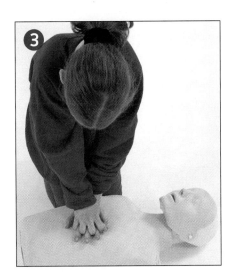

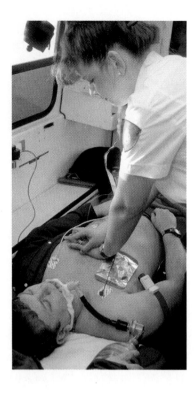

9. **Combine pressing on his chest with Rescue Breathing.**
   After pressing on his chest 15 times, tilt his head back and
   give 2 breaths of Rescue Breathing. Keep pressing 15 times
   and blowing 2 times until the Emergency Services arrive.

10. **When the Emergency Services arrive,** the trained staff will take
    over and give any specialist treatment necessary. They need to
    know exactly what has happened and what you have done so
    far. Tell them as quickly and as accurately as you can. They will
    then take your casualty to hospital where advanced medical treat-
    ment will be given.

THE EMERGENCY SERVICES

Emergency ambulances in Britain have highly trained people on board
called Paramedics. They are also fitted with special medical equipment
normally only found in hospitals. Paramedics can give hospital treatment
at the rescue scene and during the return journey. The casualty is treated
much sooner and has a much better chance of recovery.

*Rookie Tip: When you
hand the casualty over to
the paramedics tell them
everything you know
about the casualty and
the emergency, even the
smallest detail. This will
help them decide on their
treatment.*

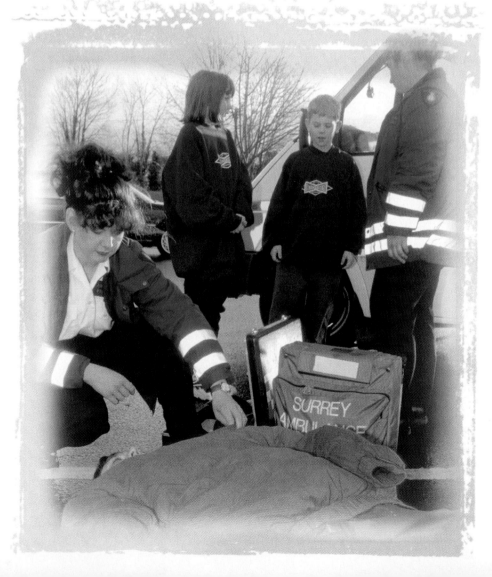

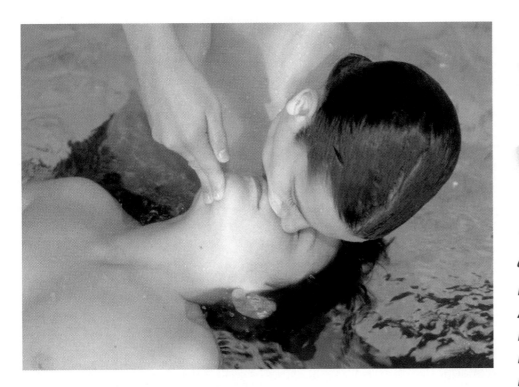

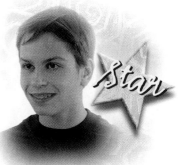

Rookie

Hi, I'm Andrew or Andy to my mates. I've got my Lifesaving 1, 2 and 3 Awards and I really enjoy my Rookie Emergency Response. Rescue Breathing in the water is fun but also quite difficult. Remember, when practising, never blow into your partner's nose.

Rescue Breathing in the Water

When you rescue someone and he is not breathing, the faster you can start Rescue Breathing the better. In the water, you blow gently into the casualty's nose, rather than his mouth.

- As soon as you reach shallow water you can begin Rescue Breathing.
- Wade, holding on to your casualty.
- Place one hand under his shoulders and with your other hand, hold his chin.
- Keep his head tilted back. Close his mouth with your fingers and seal your mouth over his nose.
- Blow gently into his nose.

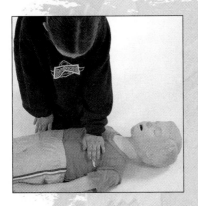

The Rescue Breathing and CPR shown in this chapter apply to casualties who are grown-ups. If the casualty is a small person or young child you should only use one hand. Do not press down as much or as hard. You only press 5 times followed by 1 breath of Rescue Breathing.

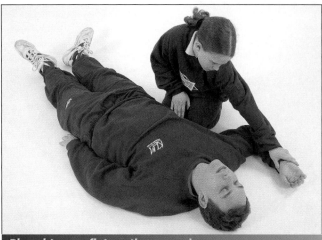

Place his arm flat on the ground

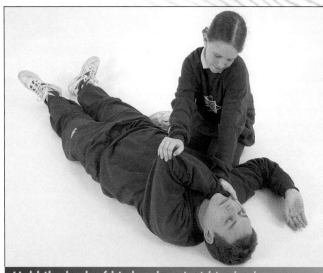

Hold the back of his hand against his cheek

THE RECOVERY POSITION

- Take the casualty's glasses off and remove anything bulky from his pockets.

- Lie him on his back with both legs straight.

- Kneel down next to him.

- Open the airway—see Rescue Breathing.

- Place his arm nearest to you flat on the ground with the elbow bent and the palm of the hand facing up.

- Bring his other arm across his chest and hold the back of his hand against his cheek.

- Raise his far knee with your other hand, keeping his foot flat on the ground.

- Pull on the knee to roll him towards you on to his side.

- Move his top leg so that both the hip and knee are level.

- Tilt back his head to make sure the airway is open.

- Keep checking his breathing and pulse.

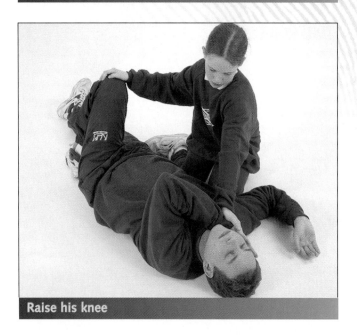

Raise his knee

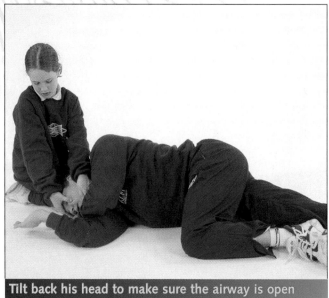

Tilt back his head to make sure the airway is open

LIFE SUPPORT TO KEEP YOUR CASUALTY ALIVE

Other types of emergency may happen where you may need to give Life Support. These are listed below. It tells you here what is wrong, how the casualty may look and feel and what you need to do to help.

Bleeding

The casualty will be bleeding from a wound. She may also be shocked, dizzy or even unconscious.

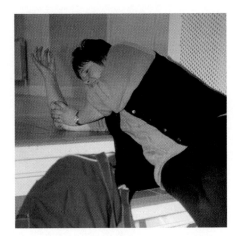

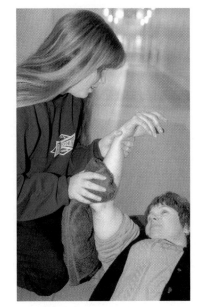

What you should do Press on the wound using a dressing or a pad of clean material. If you haven't got anything you can use, simply use your fingers or the palm of your hand. If the bleeding does not stop, apply more dressings. If nothing is available for you to use or if something is sticking out of the wound, gently and firmly press the edges together with your fingers. Lay the casualty down in a comfortable position and raise the injured part higher than the level of her chest, if you can. Treat her for shock (See page 84.) and call for a doctor.

Choking

This is when a person cannot breathe because she has something stuck in her throat.

The casualty may grip her throat with her hand, be distressed and cough with noisy wheezy breathing. If her throat is completely blocked, she may not be able to speak or even cough. Her face may start to turn blue and look frightened.

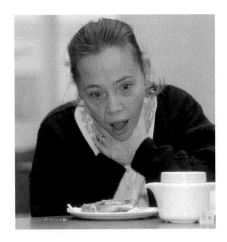

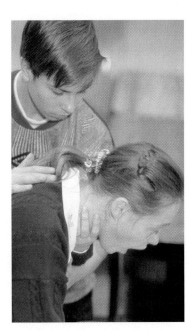

What you should do Encourage the casualty to cough. Stand to the side and slightly behind her. Support her chest with one hand and lean her forward. Give up to five sharp slaps between her shoulder blades with the heel of your other hand. Try to clear her throat with each slap. If this does not work, get help quickly.

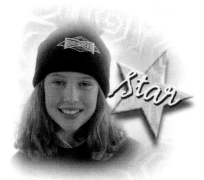

Rookie

Hi, my name is Jo and I like practising Rescue Breathing and CPR. It is good to learn all the different treatments for casualties. Maybe one day I will save someone! Can you tell me the difference between the treatment for Drowning and Bleeding?

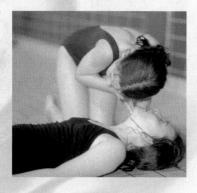

Rookie Tip: All casualties must go to hospital as breathing difficulties could start later.

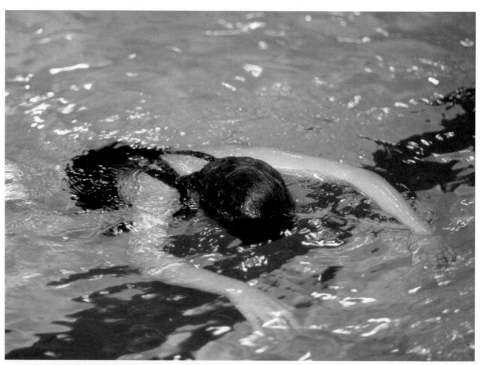

Drowning

This is when a casualty cannot breathe because her nose and mouth are underwater. She may have swallowed water.

The casualty may look lifeless. She may be unconscious and not breathing. She could be lying face down in the water, either at the surface or under the water. Her skin could look blue or grey and she could be frothing at the mouth and vomiting.

What you should do Decide whether she needs Rescue Breathing or CPR. (See page 75.) If she does, begin immediately.

Turn her over on to her back and clear away anything that is in her mouth such as seaweed. Continue CPR or Rescue Breathing even though you may think it is not making any difference. Remember it may take some time to start working especially if she has been in cold water.

Keep her as flat as possible with her feet slightly raised. This helps with shock and allows water to drain from her mouth.

Do not try to get any water out of her lungs. This is very dangerous and could result in any water in her stomach being breathed into her lungs.

If she does not need either CPR or Rescue Breathing, treat her for shock. (See page 84.)

Get her to hospital.

Heart Attack

This is an interruption to the regular heartbeat.

The casualty may feel a tightness or pain across his chest spreading to his shoulder, arm, throat or jaw. His skin may turn pale and he could be sweaty and breathless.

What you should do Immediately send for an ambulance. Loosen any tight clothing and sit him down in a comfortable position. Try to keep him as still as possible and reassure him.

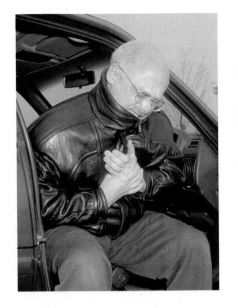

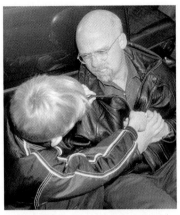

Rookie Tip: Be prepared to give CPR if his breathing and pulse stop.

Hypothermia

This is when the body's inside temperature drops so low that the body cannot warm itself up again. You should be prepared for this after a rescue from cold water or after a casualty has been exposed to cold weather.

The casualty may feel very cold to touch, particularly in her armpits. Early signs include shivering, cold and pale skin, slurring of speech, stumbling and confusion.

What you should do Lay her flat. Check her breathing and pulse and begin Rescue Breathing if necessary. Prevent her from getting any colder by putting her in a sleeping bag or cover her completely (including her head) with a blanket or spare clothing. Do not undress her. Move her out of the cold under shelter. Keep her well wrapped up so she can warm up gradually.

Rookie Tip: If she is conscious, you may give her a warm drink, but no alcohol.

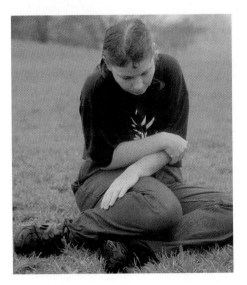

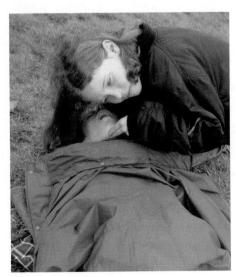

Rookie Tip: Keep the casualty warm, don't give her anything to eat or drink and get medical help quickly.

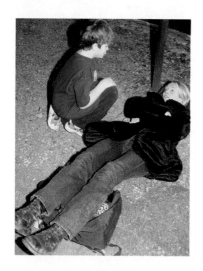

Shock

Someone goes into shock when not enough blood reaches the brain, heart and rest of the body. This should be expected after an accident such as being injured or nearly drowning.

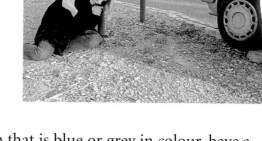

The casualty may feel faint, dizzy and confused. She may be shivering, have sweaty skin that is blue or grey in colour, have a fast heartbeat which is getting weaker and she may be breathing quickly.

What you should do Attend to the injury which may be the cause of the shock and speak reassuringly. Lay her flat on the ground with her legs raised and keep her warm. If she becomes unconscious place her in the recovery position.

Unconscious

This is where the casualty is not responding to you and is not moving. A casualty may become unconscious because of an injury or a medical condition.

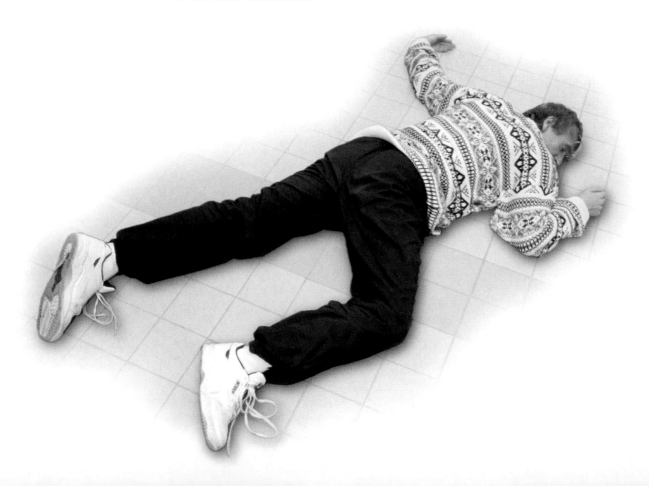

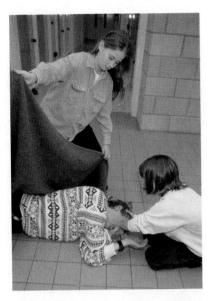

What you should do Follow your Rookie Emergency Response. (See page 75.) Check if there are any dangers and if the casualty responds. Call for help and do not move him unless you really have to. Check if his airway is open, if he is breathing and if he has got a pulse. Examine and treat any serious injuries. If he is unconscious but breathing normally place him in the recovery position. Protect him from the cold and wet and keep an eye on his breathing.

Rookie Tip: Do not leave him on his own any longer than is necessary. Do not give him anything to eat or drink.

Major Accidents with Several Casualties

With more than one casualty, always attend to the most seriously injured first. This means that you should first deal with:

1. Someone needing Rescue Breathing or CPR.
2. Someone who is choking.
3. Someone who is bleeding.
4. Someone who is unconscious and breathing.
5. Someone in shock.

What you should do To help your casualties recover you should keep them warm and dry, talk to them to calm and reassure them. Treat their injuries and keep a close eye on them. Make sure that they all get to hospital as soon as possible.

Rookies need to understand the priorities for dealing with an emergency and why it is important to call the Emergency Services as soon as possible.

FIRST AID

You may also have to deal with emergencies where a life is not in immediate danger. These may be:

- applying a triangular bandage and dressing
- asthma
- broken bones (fractures)
- epilepsy
- fainting
- hiccups
- nose bleed
- something in the eye
- sprains
- stings

You can learn how to deal with all these emergencies in the current British Red Cross, St John and St Andrew's First Aid manual.

RLSS UK Rookie— Emergency Response Certificate

The Rookie Programme includes an Emergency Response Certificate for 4 Star Grades. This can be taken either on its own or as part of other Rookie training. There are three RLSS UK Life Support Awards included in the Rookie Programme. For younger Rookies there is Junior Life Support and Rescue Breathing while older Rookies can take the Life Support 1 Award.

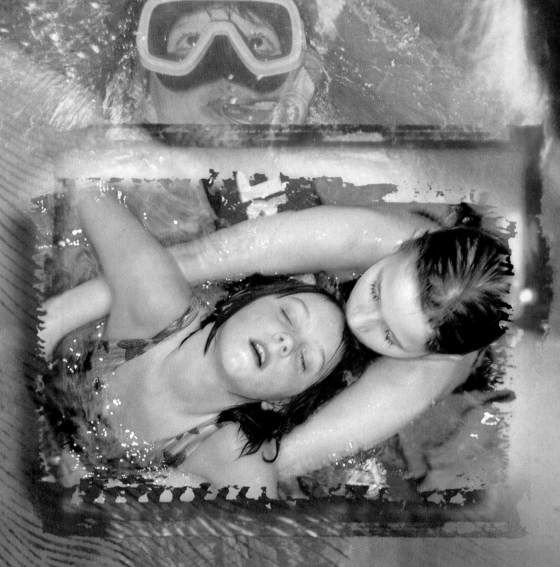

Lifeguarding and Equipment Skills

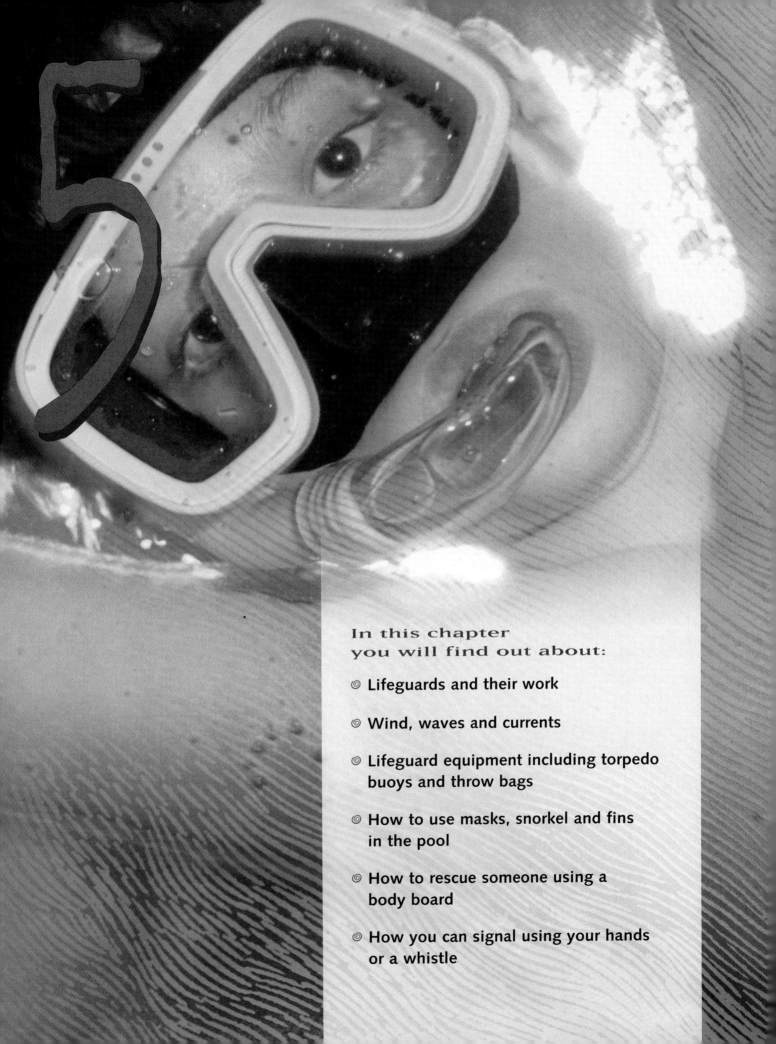

**In this chapter
you will find out about:**

◎ Lifeguards and their work

◎ Wind, waves and currents

◎ Lifeguard equipment including torpedo
  buoys and throw bags

◎ How to use masks, snorkel and fins
  in the pool

◎ How to rescue someone using a
  body board

◎ How you can signal using your hands
  or a whistle

*F*inding out about the skills and equipment used by Pool and Beach Lifeguards is fun. In this chapter you will learn about all the special rescue equipment used by Lifeguards. You can use all this equipment, except for rescue boards and rescue skis, in a swimming pool—but ask permission first.

This chapter has two parts. The first part tells you about the skills. The second part, "Now You Try it!" shows you how to practise the skills. Have fun!

LIFEGUARDS

Lifeguards are trained to keep people safe by preventing accidents and dealing with emergencies.

Lifeguards:

• Encourage people to behave in a safe and responsible way when they are near or in water.

• Prevent people from getting into difficulties.

• Give advice on pool and beach safety.

Rookie Tip: Remember, as a Rookie you are learning to be a lifesaver but not a lifeguard.

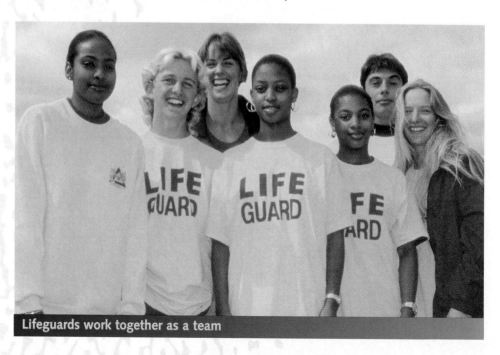

Lifeguards work together as a team

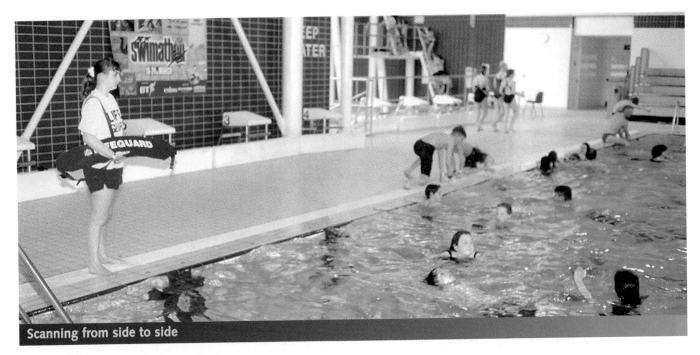

Scanning from side to side

- Supervise the pool or beach all the time.
- Carry out rescues using special rescue equipment.
- Give immediate First Aid and aftercare.

Areas supervised by lifeguards are called Patrol Zones or Patrol Areas. Beach Patrol Zones or Areas are marked with red and yellow flags. In these areas, lifeguards watch the water looking from side to side to make sure they can see anybody who may be in difficulty. This is called scanning.

A group of lifeguards works together as a team. By working together the group makes sure:

- There is always one lifeguard scanning while the others relax.
- One lifeguard can go for help while the others make a rescue.
- They can all help each other.

Rookie Tip: Practice working together with other Rookies when you rescue someone.

Uniform The international colours for lifeguards are red and yellow and they usually wear red shorts and a yellow top. Beach lifeguards also wear long-sleeved tops and wide brimmed hats to protect them from the sun.

Lifeguards and lifesavers There is a difference between lifeguards and lifesavers.

A lifeguard is someone whose job is to prevent accidents and save people who are in trouble.

A lifesaver is a person who has been trained to save lives.

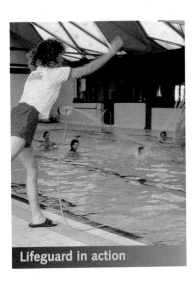

Lifeguard in action

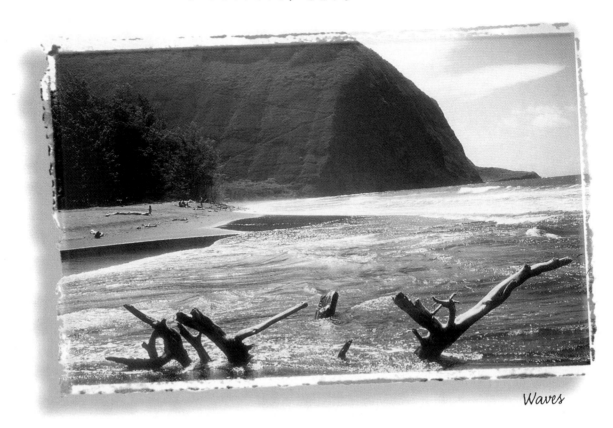

Waves

SEA AWARENESS

The beach is a very different place from a swimming pool and it is important that you understand the dangers there. Always remember that the water is very powerful and can easily hurt you.

Winds

Rookie Tip: Never chase after inflatables or balls that an offshore wind is blowing out to sea.

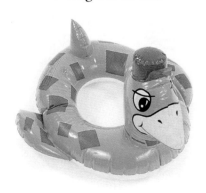

Onshore winds These blow from the sea on to the shore. They can make the waves so much more powerful that they become dangerous.

Offshore winds These blow from the shore out to sea. Remember that although the water near to the shore may be calm, an offshore wind can make the sea very dangerous further out. Offshore winds can blow inflatables and wind surfers away from the shore.

You can find out if there is an offshore or onshore wind by looking at which way any flags are flying or you can hold something up to be blown by the wind such as a handkerchief or T-shirt.

Waves

Waves can be fun but are also dangerous. When the wind blows across the sea it makes waves. These can be different in size and type, it all depends on how strong the wind is, how long it has been blowing, where it has come from and how deep the water is. The sea can still have waves on it even after the wind has died down.

Dumping waves These break with huge force. They can be dangerous as a swimmer can be thrown to the bottom and dragged out to sea by the water when it rushes back out.

Spilling waves These are waves with a crest of surf tumbling down the front. They are the best waves for body surfers, swimmers and board riders.

Surging waves You find these on very deep water. They are very powerful and can knock you off your feet or even pluck you from the shoreline.

Swimming in unbroken waves is not a problem although it can be a bit murky. Do this if a wave seems likely to crash down on you.

- Breath in and surface dive to lie on the bottom just before the wave arrives.
- Dig your fingers in the sand and hold on to the bottom with both hands.
- Place your feet on the bottom.
- Push off towards the surface on the seaward side of the wave.

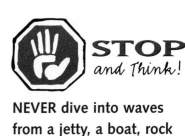

Dumping Wave

Spilling Wave

Surging Wave

Types of waves

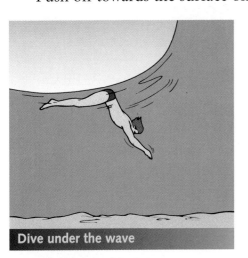

Dive under the wave

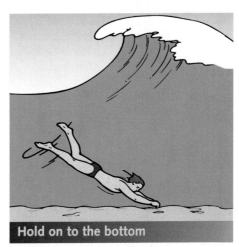

Hold on to the bottom

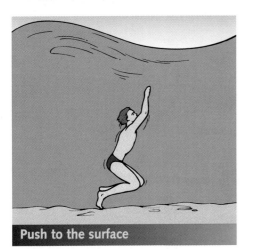

Push to the surface

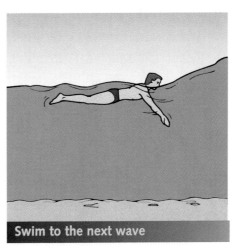

Swim to the next wave

STOP *and Think!*

NEVER dive into waves from a jetty, a boat, rock cliffs or the poolside. If in doubt, ask the lifeguard.

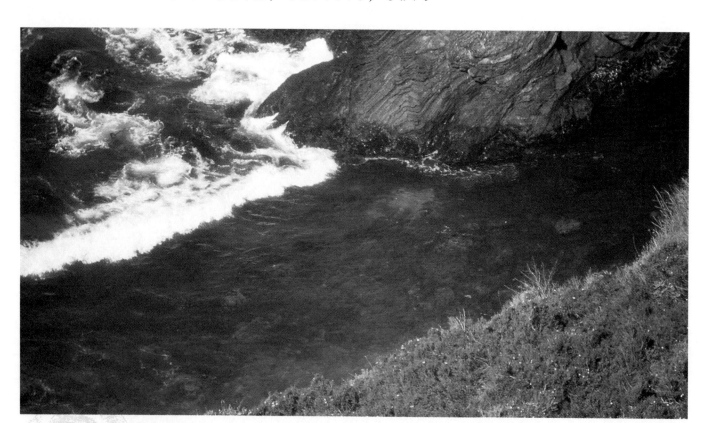

Currents

Sea currents are caused by tides and waves.

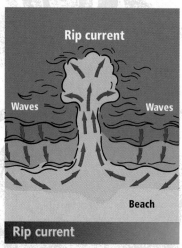

Rip current

Rip current This is where all the water coming in on to the beach makes channels along the beach before running back out to sea. A rip current is very dangerous. It can be very strong and even powerful swimmers may not be able to swim against it. Remember, the bigger the waves are, the stronger the current will be.

A rip current can be recognised by:

- Discoloured water—usually brown foam on the surface beyond the breaking waves.
- Debris floating back to sea with the current.
- Where there is surf, a rip current will make the waves smaller.

Rookies should be able to describe how waves are formed, different wave types and a rip current. They should also be able to explain how to swim through waves and about the dangers of currents.

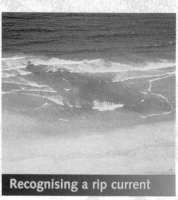

Recognising a rip current

RLSS UK Rookie—Ocean Awareness Certificate

The Rookie Programme includes an Ocean Awareness Certificate, this includes Rescue Principles which is about the work of a Lifeguard and Sea Awareness.

LIFEGUARD EQUIPMENT

Torpedo Buoy (Rescue Tube)

Also known as a Peterson Tube. These are foam filled flexible floating supports. They are bright red with a shoulder strap and can be carried by the lifeguard. Torpedo buoys can be used for most rescues. They can support three to five casualties or be clipped around an unconscious casualty. You can carry it in your hand or keep it handy in a boat or next to the lifeguard observation post.

Knots

Ropes are used to make rescues, stow away equipment and for First Aid. You need to know which knot to use when, and how to tie it.

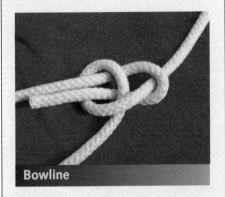

Bowline

This knot is used to make a loop at the end of a rope which will not slip but which can be untied easily.

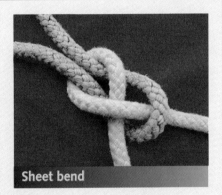

Sheet bend

This knot is used to tie together two ropes of a different thickness.

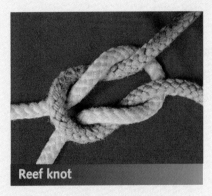

Reef knot

This knot is used in First Aid as it is flat. It can be untied easily.

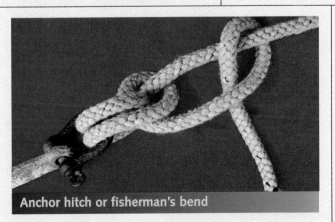

Anchor hitch or fisherman's bend

This knot is used to tie a rope to an anchor.

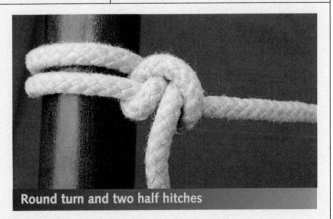

Round turn and two half hitches

This knot is used to tie a boat securely to a post or a mooring ring.

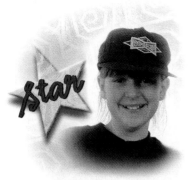

Rookie

Hi, my name is Amelia. One of the best things in Rookie is to use the lifeguard equipment and the throw bag is my favourite. I am learning to hit a target 10 metres away. If you can borrow a throw bag, you try it.

Coiling a Rope

When you coil a rope, you make a lot of loops that lie next to each other. To do this, you hold one end in one hand and stretch your arms apart to get two arm lengths of rope. You then take the place that you are holding and put it in the other hand. You need to twist your wrist as you do this to make the rope lie flat. Repeat this until the rope is neatly coiled.

Throw Bag

This is a small bright red fabric bag with yellow throwing line coiled up inside. When you throw the bag the line uncoils. This is a very quick and easy to use rescue aid.

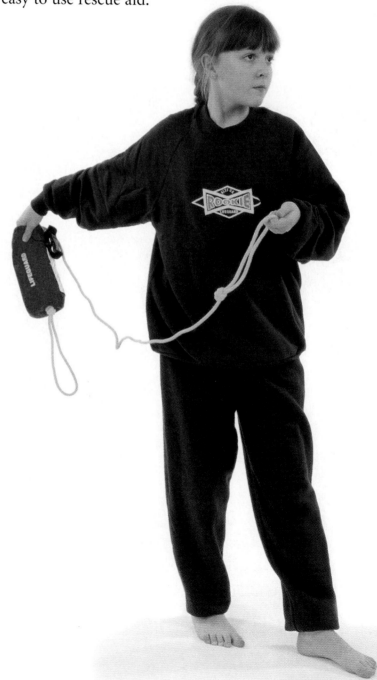

RLSS UK Rookie— Equipment Certificate

The Rookie Programme includes an Equipment Certificate. To get this you need to know about Torpedo Buoys, Knots and Throw Bags.

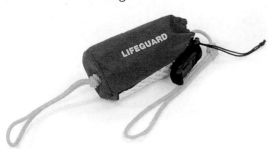

MASK, SNORKEL AND FINS

Mask, snorkel and fins are great fun to use because they let you see, breathe and swim when your face is down under the water. Always try them in the pool first time and make sure that you ask the lifeguard before using them.

Mask

A mask makes a water tight air pocket around your eyes and nose so that you can see under the water. It has a silicone or rubber frame with a strap and shatterproof glass window.

Choosing a mask Faces and masks are all very different in shape and size so you need to find a mask that fits you well. To find the perfect fit, hold the mask in your hand and place it on your face without fitting the strap. Breathe in gently through your nose and take your hand away. If the mask stays where it is, it fits you. Choose a mask where the rubber is moulded around your nose. It is not a good idea to buy a mask with a snorkel already fitted to it. You should wash a new mask with detergent before you use it.

Rookie Tip: Always practise using your mask, snorkel and fins in the swimming pool, before you try them in open water. It is much safer.

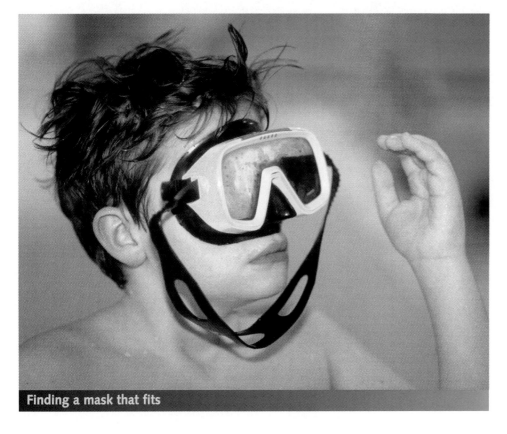
Finding a mask that fits

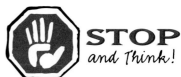

STOP *and Think!*

YOU SHOULD NOT use a mask, snorkel or fins to depths of more than 1.5 metres or when there are waves on the water.

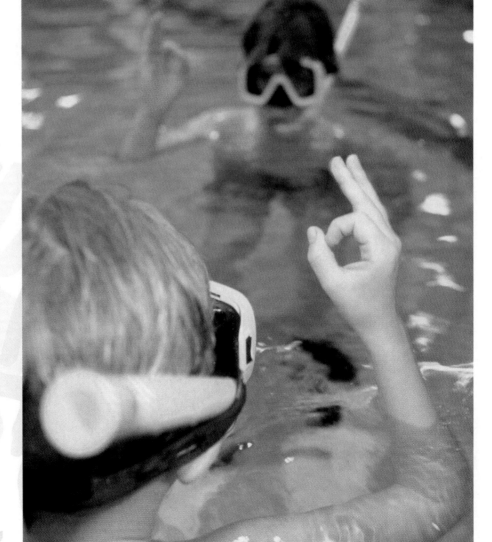

Snorkel

A snorkel is a hollow plastic tube which you can breath through as you swim with your face down under the water. It is made up of two parts, the mouthpiece and the tube. When you use it, you put the mouthpiece in your mouth behind your lips and grip it with your teeth.

Choosing a snorkel There are different types of snorkels but you should use one with an open end. Make sure that the tube is not too long, otherwise you could find yourself breathing in the stale air you have just breathed out. The snorkel should also be able to bend so it will not break and hurt you.

Safety Hand Signal

When you are wearing a snorkel and a mask you can't talk to anyone, so you need to get into the habit of signalling that everything is OK. Make a circle with your forefinger and thumb and hold it up. When your trainer or another Rookie makes this signal to you, they are asking "Are you OK?". You should make the same signal back to say, "I am OK".

Clearing your ears

Sometimes your ears can hurt when you go underwater. To stop this from happening, pinch your nose, close your mouth and gently try to blow air out of your nose. Your ears should go POP immediately. If they don't POP or if they still hurt, swim up to the surface immediately.

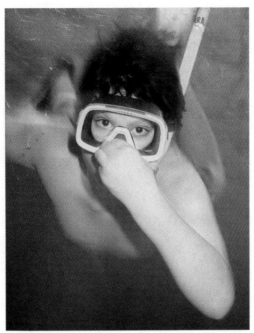

Fins

Fins make your leg action stronger and make you swim faster.

Choosing fins Fins come in different shapes and there are two types of fitting. Slipper fins fit like a shoe while open back fins are strapped to your feet. You should choose a pair which fit your feet well. Slipper fins are the most suitable to use in a swimming pool.

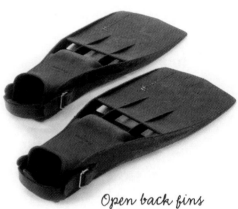

Open back fins

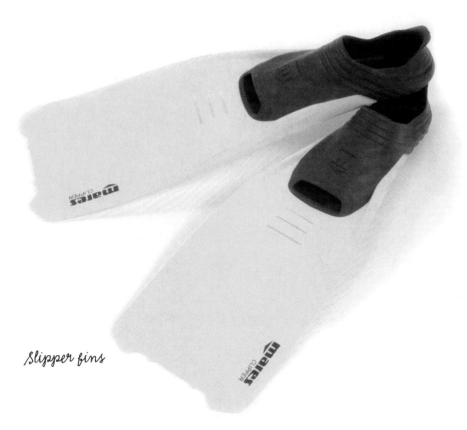

Slipper fins

RLSS UK Rookie— Snorkelling Certificate

The Rookie Programme includes a Snorkelling Certificate which involves using a Mask, Snorkel and Fins. If you want to use this equipment for diving and extended swimming underwater you need to join a special diving club and receive specialist training. See Appendix—The British Sub-Aqua Club.

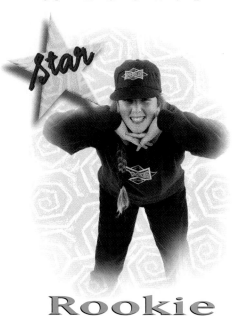

Rookie

*H*i, I'm Pia and I am a Rookie with Rushmoor Voluntary Lifeguard Club. The best thing about being a Rookie is when we use the body boards. It was difficult to balance the first time I tried it, but I'm getting better. Soon I'm going to be able to use the rescue board.

RLSS UK Rookie— Paddle Craft Certificate

The Rookie Programme includes a Paddle Craft Certificate you can get when you can use Body Boards, Rescue Skis and Rescue Boards.

PADDLE CRAFT

Body Board

Sometimes called a Boogie Board, these short body boards are used for body surfing and are a good introduction to using a full size surf board. Like the full size rescue board, the body board can also be used to make rescues.

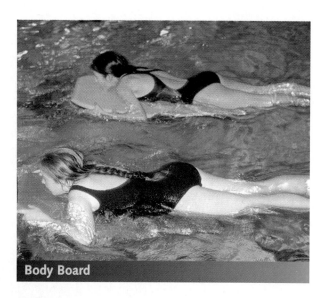
Body Board

Rescue Ski

A rescue ski is a special type of surf board with a place to sit and for your legs. It is paddled with a double ended paddle. With this, you can reach a casualty quickly and keep her afloat. The ski can be used for Rescue Breathing and for bringing a casualty to shore. Rescue skis often have grab handles attached.

Rescue Board

This is a surf board especially made for making rescues. It is some times called a Malibu Board. You can kneel or lie flat on the board and paddle it with your hands.

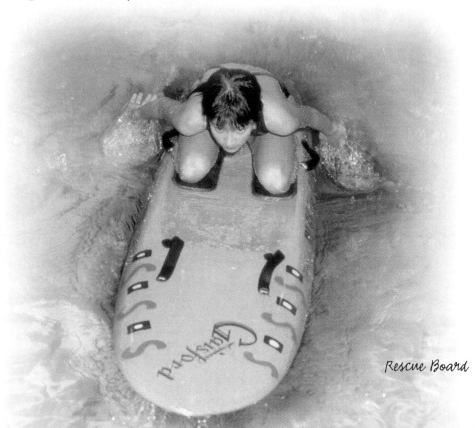
Rescue Board

SIGNALS

Sometimes you need to communicate with someone so far away that they cannot hear you. If this happens you need to use different signals. Here are some you can practise.

Hand Signals

There are different hand signals for when you are on land and when you are in the water.

When you are on land

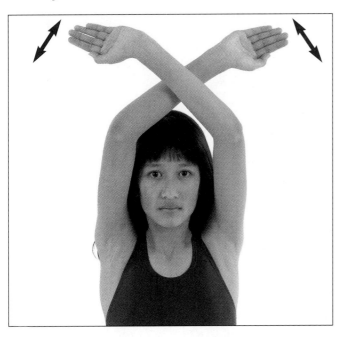

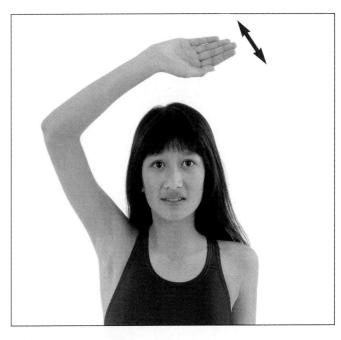

To attract attention—arms waved to and fro, crossing above the head.

Repeat message not clear—one arm waved to and fro above the head.

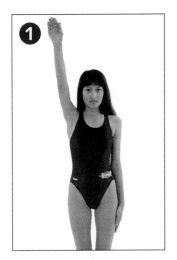
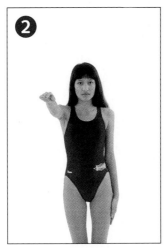
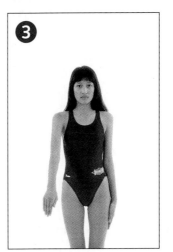
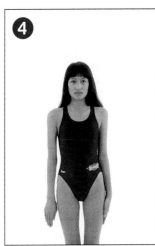

Message understood—one hand held above the head and then swept down.

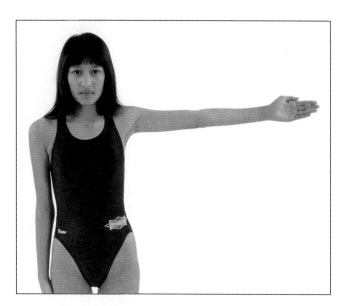 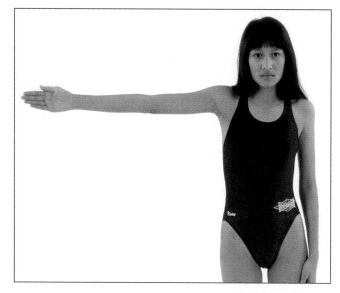

Move to the left or right—one arm out to the side.

Investigate object in the water—
arms held at 45 degrees.

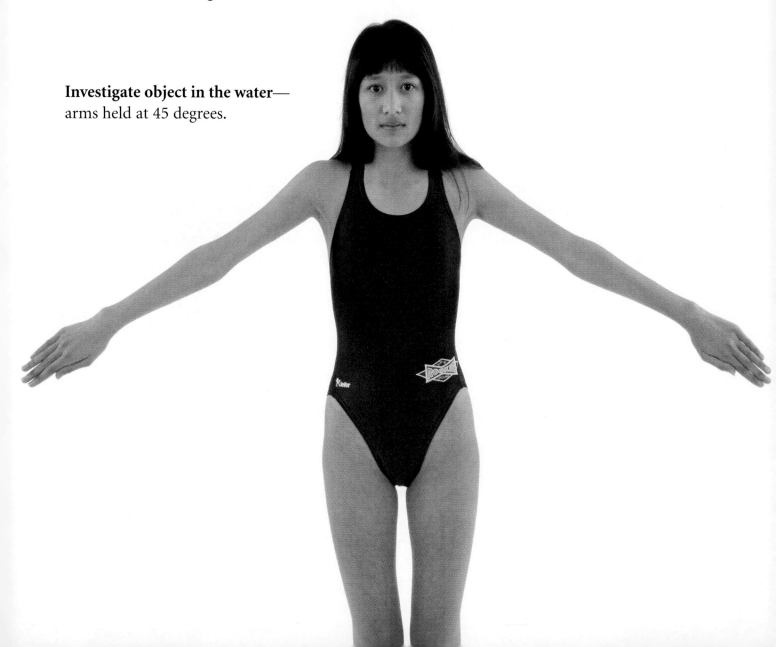

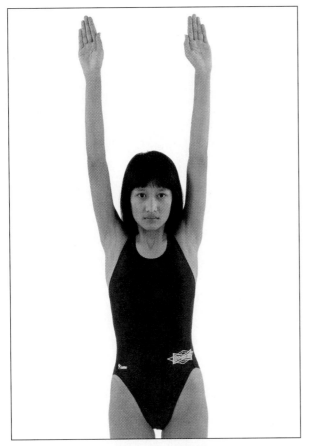

Go further out to sea—both arms straight up in the air.

Return to shore—one arm in the air.

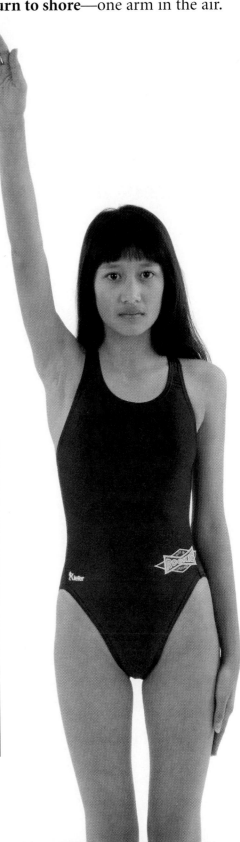

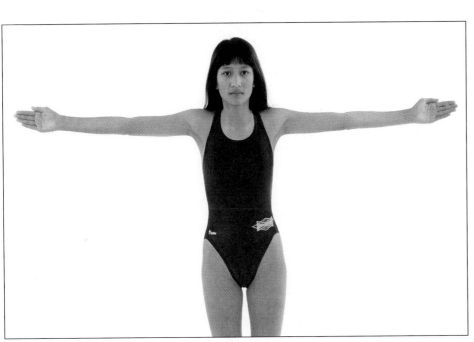

Keep still—arms outstretched to the side.

When you are in the water

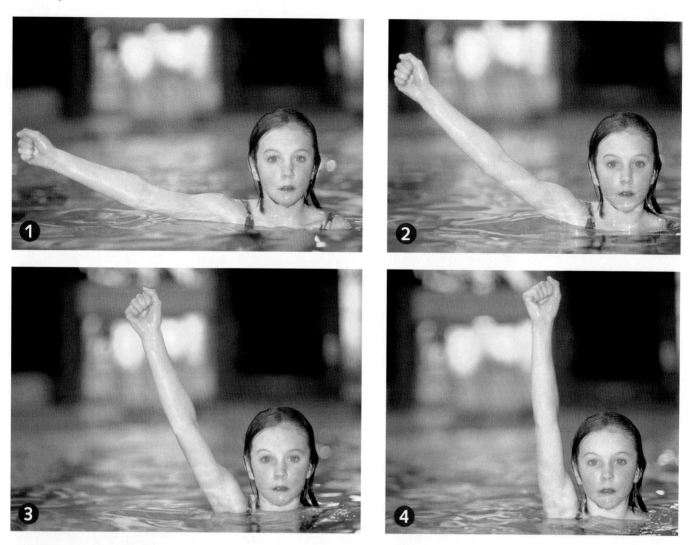

Assistance required—one arm waved to and fro above the head.

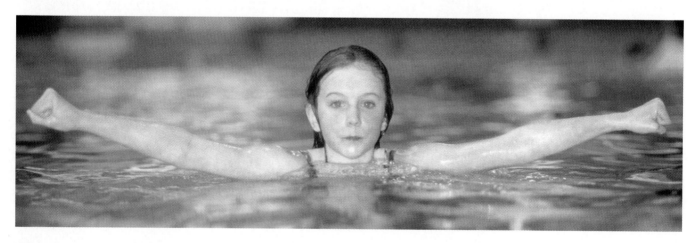

The situation is OK. All clear—both arms outstretched.

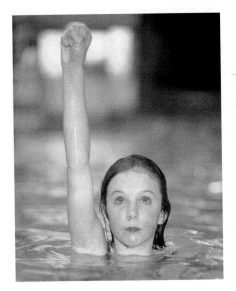

Whistle Signals
- **One short blast**
  to attract the attention of a member of the public
- **Two short blasts**
  to gain another lifeguard's attention
- **Three short blasts**
  to indicate that a lifeguard is taking emergency action

Repeat, message not clear— one arm in the air.

CUSTOMER RELATIONS

Lifeguards sometimes need to say something to members of the public to prevent a dangerous situation developing. This is called customer relations and can be quite difficult as people may not like being told what they can and can't do.

When a lifeguard has to tell someone to do something he should tell them why he wants them to do it. For example rather than saying "Don't dive there!" say "It is much safer to dive over there in deeper water."

One of the things a lifeguard sometimes has to be able to do is to read a persons body language. Body language is where you can look at someone's body and see how he feels. Lifeguards sometimes need to recognize a person who is frightened, angry, alarmed or in trouble. For example a parent looking worried and running up and down the beach may have lost a child. However, it is not enough to look at someone's body language, the lifeguard will still need to talk to him.

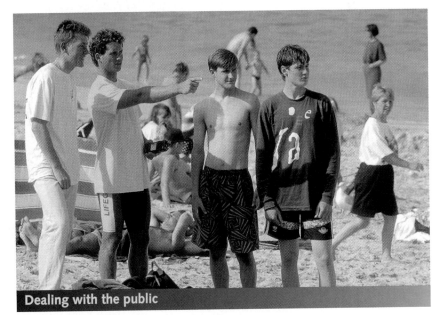

Dealing with the public

RADIOS

Radios are used on the beach to communicate between lifeguards, inshore rescue boats and the control centre. Some large indoor leisure centres also use radios to enable lifeguards to communicate with each other.

A beach lifeguard normally uses CB (Citizen Band) with a transmitting frequency of 27 MHz (Megahertz) or VHF (Very High Frequency) with a frequency band of 30-300 MHz.

There are set procedures for using and speaking on the radio called RT (Radio Telephony). These include using different channels or frequencies, saying things in the right order, using call signs and special words that indicate you are in danger such as Pan and Mayday.

Even when speaking slowly it can be difficult to understand a radio message. It may be faint, distorted and hard to hear. To overcome this, words can be spelt out using the phonetic alphabet. Each letter is given a word which is much easier to hear and avoids confusion.

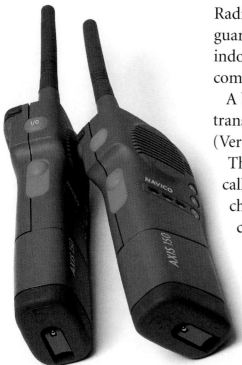

Rookie Tip: In Britain you need a special licence to use a radio.

RLSS UK Rookie— Communications Certificate

The Rookie Programme includes a Communications Certificate for Signals, Customer Relations and Radios.

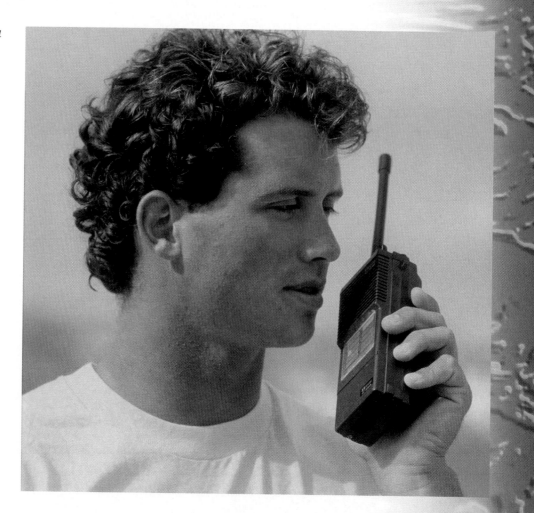

Phonetic Alphabet

A	Alpha	**N**	November
B	Bravo	**O**	Oscar
C	Charlie	**P**	Papa
D	Delta	**Q**	Quebec
E	Echo	**R**	Romeo
F	Foxtrot	**S**	Sierra
G	Golf	**T**	Tango
H	Hotel	**U**	Uniform
I	India	**V**	Victor
J	Juliet	**W**	Whisky
K	Kilo	**X**	X-ray
L	Lima	**Y**	Yankee
M	Mike	**Z**	Zulu

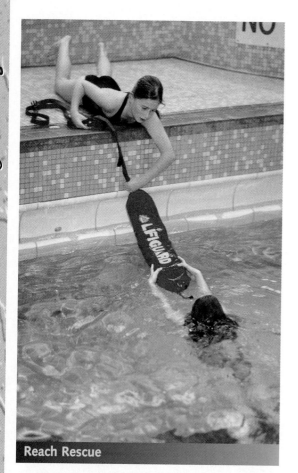

Reach Rescue

Lifeguard Equipment

Using a Torpedo Buoy

■ *Reach Rescue*

Unclip the strap and hold the end in your spare hand (not your throwing hand). Stand safely, hold the buoy lengthways in your throwing hand and throw it forward from your shoulder. Tell your partner to hold it with two hands. Lie down and pull her to safety.

■ *Throw Rescue*

Leave the shoulder strap clipped together or wrap it around the torpedo buoy. Stand safely, hold the torpedo buoy lengthways and throw it forward from your shoulder. Tell your partner to hold it with two hands and kick to safety. An alternative way is to throw the torpedo buoy either underarm or like a spear. You should practice and decide which is the best way for you.

▣ *Enter the pool with a torpedo buoy*

Put on the shoulder strap and get into the water using a Slide-in Entry. As you enter the water, throw the torpedo buoy behind you. Make sure you don't get tangled up in the strap!

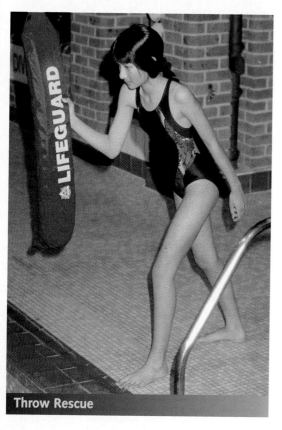

Throw Rescue

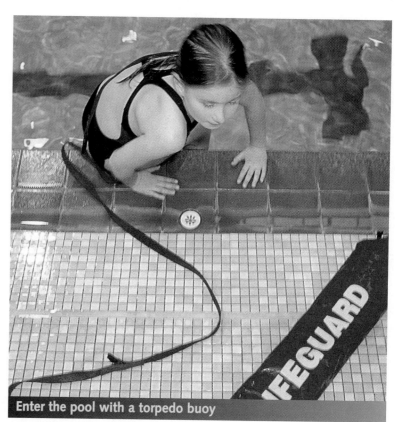

Enter the pool with a torpedo buoy

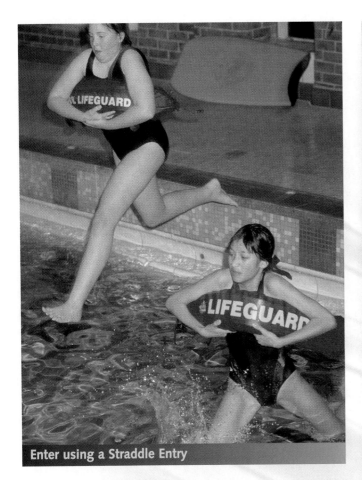

Enter using a Straddle Entry

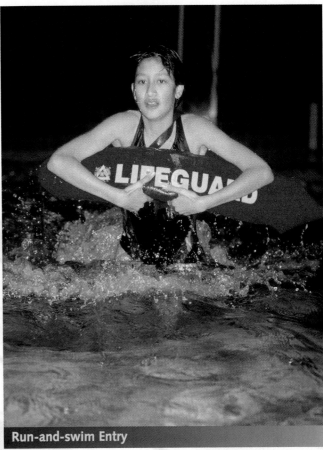

Run-and-swim Entry

Now You Try It!

■ *Enter using a Straddle Entry*

Hold the torpedo buoy across your chest with the ends under your arms. Hold the shoulder strap in your hands. For the Straddle Entry see page 29.

■ *Run-and-swim Entry from a gradual slope*

To enter the water from a gradual slope such as a wave pool or into flat water.

You can do this in one of two ways, after putting on the shoulder strap.

- Hold the torpedo buoy across your chest. Run into the water lifting your legs to avoid falling. (Do not run on the poolside.) When you cannot run any further, lean forward on to the torpedo buoy and start swimming keeping it under your arms. Do not dive into the water—this is dangerous. Use this way for making a rescue over a short distance. It should not be used when running into surf.

- Run into the water lifting your legs to avoid falling over. Hold the torpedo buoy under one arm until it is deep enough to swim, then throw the buoy a little to one side and swim towing it behind you.

Rookie Tip: When getting into the water with a torpedo buoy always make sure that you do not get tangled up in the harness.

▢ **Shallow Water**
■ **Deep Water**

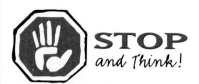

STOP
and Think!

DON'T THROW the torpedo buoy! Always pass or float it from the water.

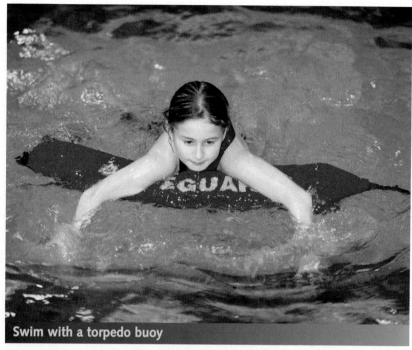

Swim with a torpedo buoy

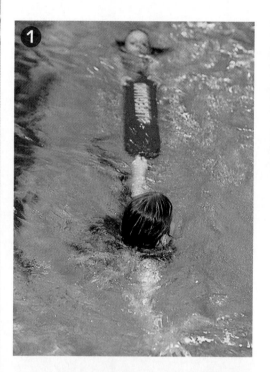

■ Swim with a torpedo buoy

Begin by placing the shoulder strap across your shoulder.

For rescues with a short swim to your partner, you should use Front Crawl or Breast Stroke with the torpedo buoy across your chest and under your arms.

For rescues with a long swim to your partner, you should swim, towing it behind you, with the strap over your head and across your chest.

■ Rescue a conscious casualty

Swim to your partner. Move the shoulder strap over your head so that it is only over one shoulder. Reach out with the torpedo buoy and tell her to lean forward, grab it and kick her legs. You hold the other end of the torpedo buoy and tow your partner to safety. Make sure you don't get too close in case she grabs you (1).

Now try it with your partner lying on her back and holding the torpedo buoy lengthways down her chest. Make sure that the strap end of the torpedo buoy is pointing over her shoulder (2).

■ Support Position with a torpedo buoy

Put your partner in the Support Position (See page 71.) with the torpedo buoy across your chest and under your arms.

Rookie Tip: When you are towing a casualty make sure you can let go of the torpedo buoy easily.

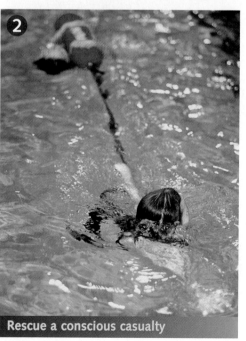

Rescue a conscious casualty

Support Position with a torpedo buoy

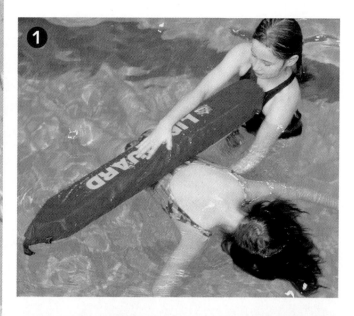

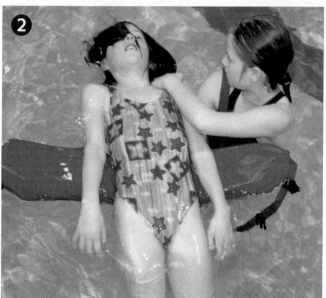

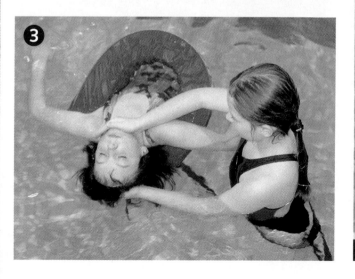

■ *Turn an unconscious casualty on to her back*

You can do this one of two ways.

- Slide the torpedo buoy under the chest of your partner. Clip the buoy together across her back and turn her on to her back.
- Place the torpedo buoy over the bottom of her back and hold it in place with one hand (1). Hold her chest or shoulder with the other hand, turn her on to her back with the torpedo buoy underneath her (2). Clip the buoy around her. Turn the torpedo buoy so that it is over her chest (3).

■ *Tow an unconscious casualty*

Ask your partner to pretend she is unconscious. Clip the torpedo buoy around her with the shoulder strap extended. Swim Side Stroke or Lifesaving Backstroke and at the same time keep watching your partner.

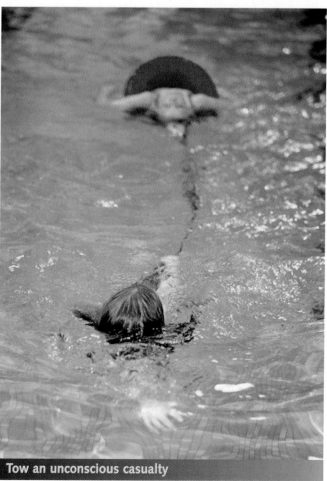

Tow an unconscious casualty

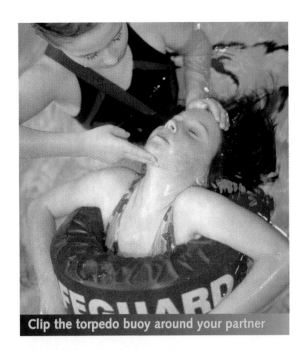

Clip the torpedo buoy around your partner

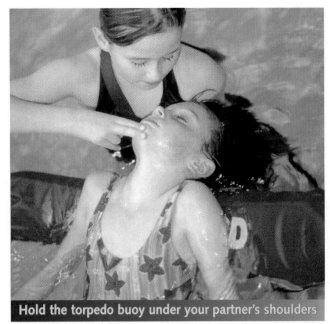

Hold the torpedo buoy under your partner's shoulders

Now You Try It!

Give rescue breathing while wading

You can do Rescue Breathing in the water (See page 79.)
in two ways.

- Clip the torpedo buoy around your partner making sure that the clip is on her chest.
- Hold the torpedo buoy under your partner's shoulders.

Using a Throw Bag

Open the bag wide and hold the loop of the throwing rope in one
hand. Hold the neck of the bag with your throwing hand. Stand back
from the edge and throw the bag underarm, keeping your throwing
arm straight. Let go just before your arm is level with your shoulder.

*Rookie Tip: When you repack
a throw bag you should feed
the rope carefully back into the
bag so that it does not snag.*

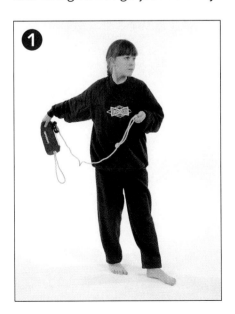

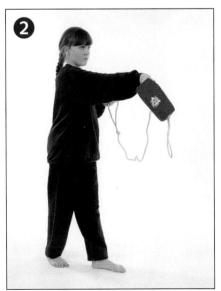

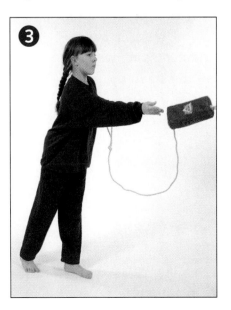

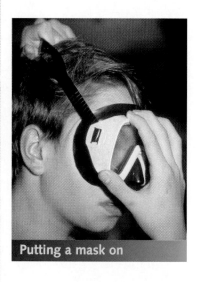

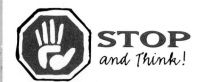
Putting a mask on

Rookie Tip: Always hold the mask against your face when you fit or remove the strap.

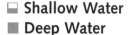**STOP** *and Think!*

WHEN YOU USE your fins, snorkel and mask for the first time, start off in shallow water in the swimming pool where you can stand up.

☐ **Shallow Water**
■ **Deep Water**

Using Mask, Snorkel and Fins

Make sure that you can clear your mask and snorkel before your start finning.

Putting a mask on and taking it off

To stop the mask from misting up, spit into it, wipe around the window and wash it out. Brush the hair away from your forehead and wet your face. Hold the mask on your face while you fit or remove the strap. Make sure the strap is not too tight.

☐ *Clearing mask under water*

Kneel on the bottom of the pool with your face just under the water. Tilt your head back to look up and place two fingers in the middle of the top edge of the mask (1). Press the top edge against your forehead and blow out hard through your nose (2). This will force the water out.

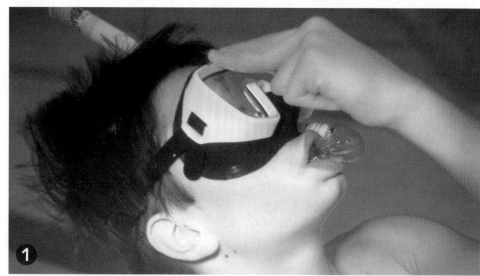

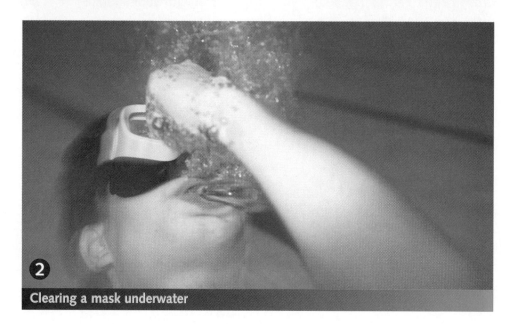
Clearing a mask underwater

Putting a snorkel on

Place the tube under the strap of your mask and put the mouthpiece in your mouth. Breathe in slowly, then breathe out with more force.

Clearing your snorkel

When you dive down under the water your snorkel tube will fill with water. When you get to the surface clear it by blowing sharply to force the water out. You can also tilt your head back and let the water drain out. The next breath you take should be small otherwise you may breathe in the water left in the snorkel.

Rookie Tip: When you are snorkelling, the tube should be pointing straight up.

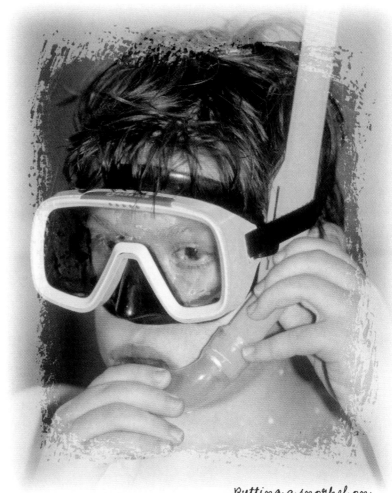

putting a snorkel on

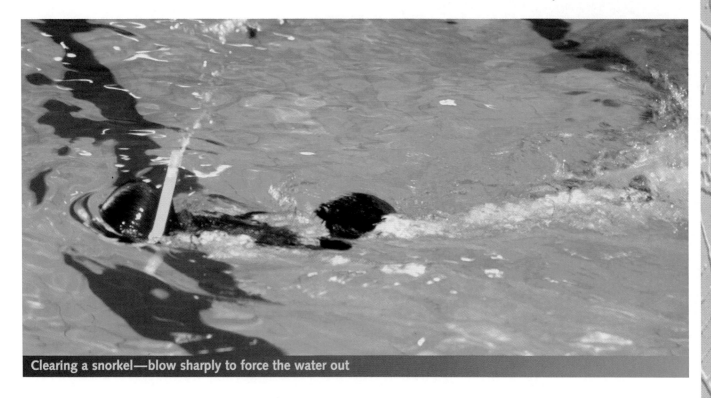

Clearing a snorkel—blow sharply to force the water out

Now You Try It!

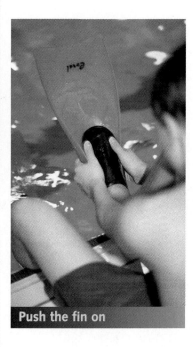

Push the fin on

Rookie Tip: Never go snorkelling on your own, always go with a friend.

Putting fins on

Push the fin on your foot rather than pull it from the heel.

Walking in fins

Always walk backwards or sideways. If you need to go up or down steps, take the fins off and put them back on in the water.

Finning

When you kick your legs, point your toes and keep your ankles loose and floppy. Kick slowly and keep your arms loose down the side of your body.

You can kick your legs in two ways.

- Kick you legs up and down alternately as if you are swimming Front Crawl.
- Keep your legs together while you kick them up and down. This is known as the Dolphin Kick.

Snorkelling

Fit your mask, snorkel and fins carefully and check they are on properly. Before you get into the water, place the mask on your forehead with two hands. When you are in the water, place the mask on your face. Put your face down in the water and breathe through your snorkel. Start finning up and down at the side of the pool. Now try finning across shallow water with your arms by your sides.

Dolphin Kick

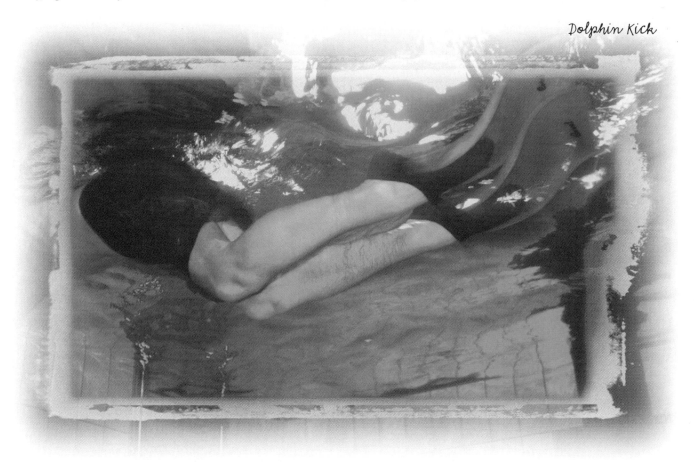

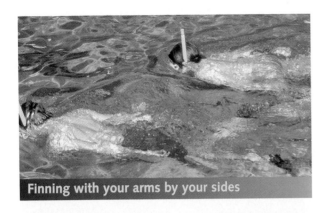
Finning with your arms by your sides

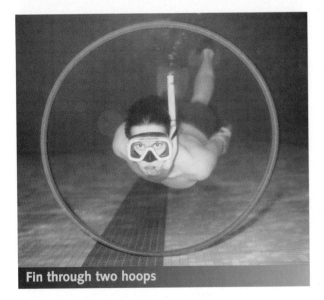
Fin through two hoops

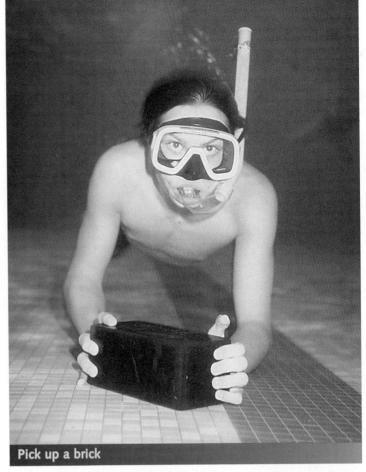
Pick up a brick

When you can do this confidently you can also try these skills:

- Fin on your front, side and back.
- Dive below the surface and clear your ears and your snorkel.
- Dive below the surface and clear your mask.
- Dive to the bottom of the pool, no deeper than 1.5 metres and fin through two hoops.
- Do a forward and backward roll underwater.
- Dive to the bottom, no deeper than 1.5 metres and bring something up to the surface, such as a brick.
- Dive to the bottom, no deeper than 1.5 metres and bring up a submersed manikin. (Use both hands to pick up the manikin.)
- Tow an unconscious casualty. (Ask your partner to pretend she is unconscious.)

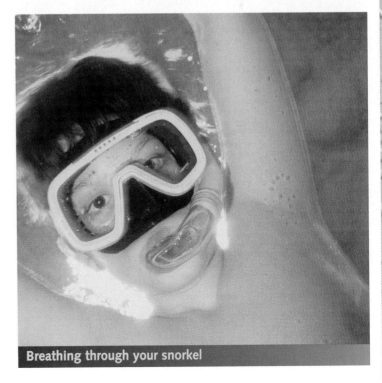
Breathing through your snorkel

Now You Try It!

◻ **Shallow Water**
◼ **Deep Water**

Paddle Craft

Using a Body Board

◼ *Getting on the board*

Push off and slide on to the middle of the board. Move your body to find the best place to balance your board, remembering that it should be slightly up at the nose. Too far forward, the front will dig in.
Too far back and it will create resistance.

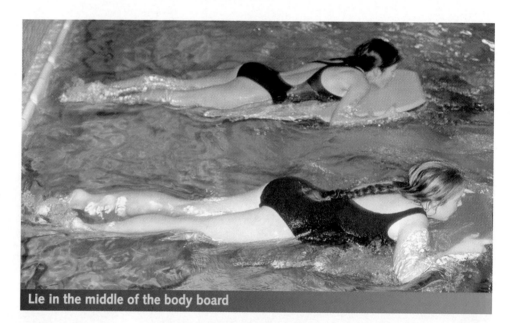

Lie in the middle of the body board

Rookie Tip: When you have found the best balancing position, remember where your chin is on the board. If your chin is in the same place each time, the rest of your body will be perfectly balanced.

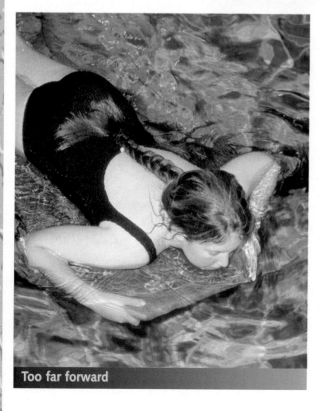

Too far forward

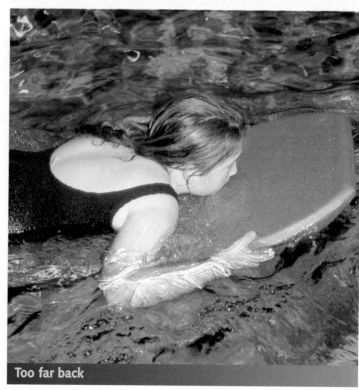

Too far back

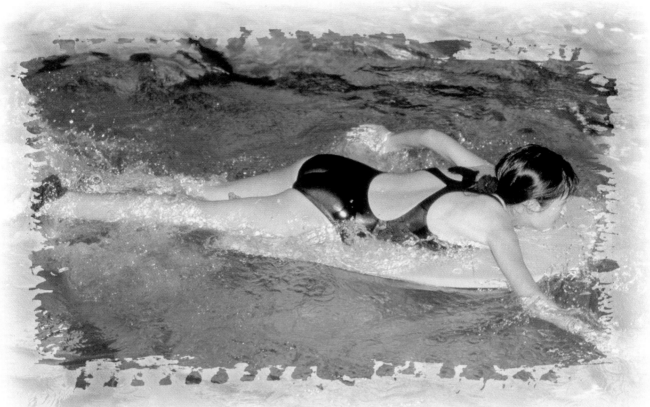

Paddling—use Front Crawl arms and legs

Paddling

Use Front Crawl arms and legs. A pair of fins will make you go faster. To steer, drag a foot in the water on the side you wish to turn and paddle harder with the opposite arm.

If you are only using your legs to kick, hold on to each side of the board about six inches from the leading edge.

Paddling in waves

To go through waves paddle straight at them. If a wave is about to break on top of you roll the board so the wave hits the bottom of the board—not you.

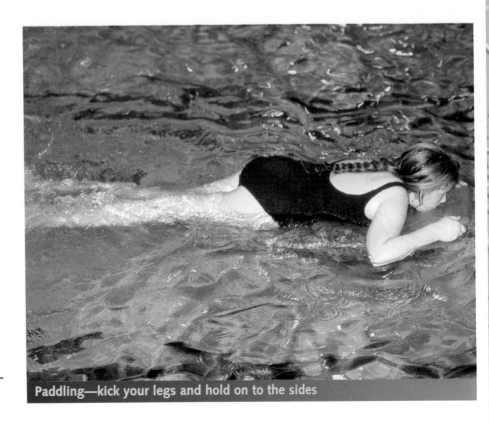

Paddling—kick your legs and hold on to the sides

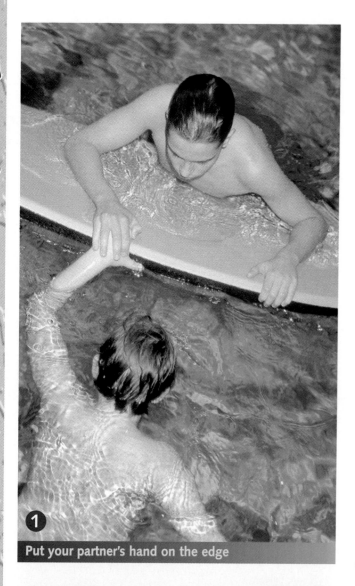

1 Put your partner's hand on the edge

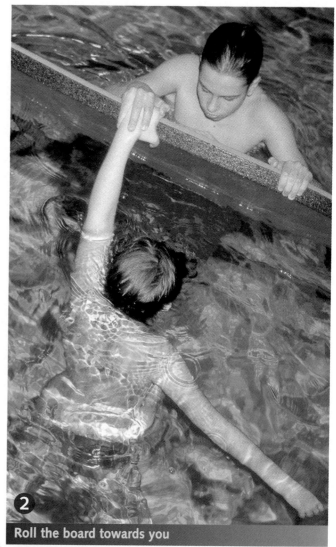

2 Roll the board towards you

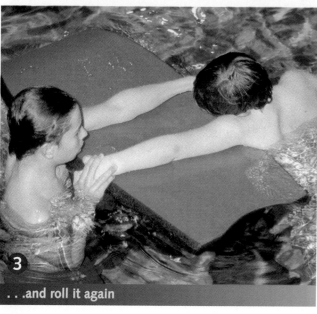

3 . . .and roll it again

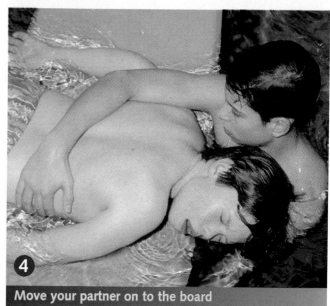

4 Move your partner on to the board

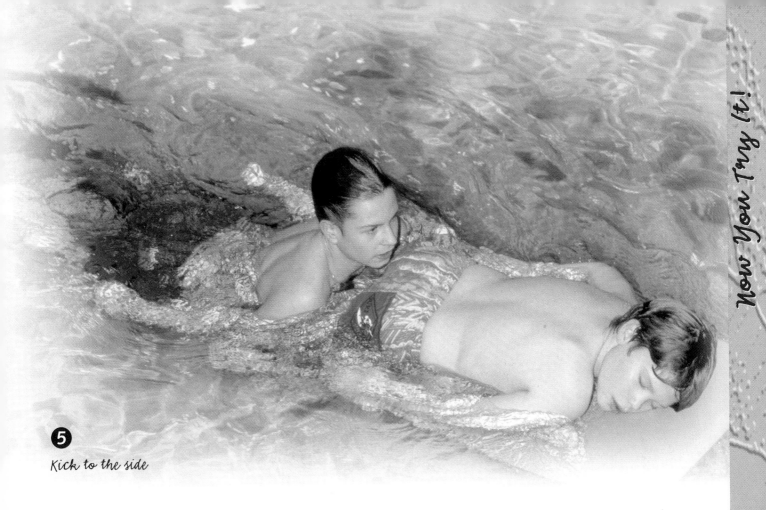

5

Kick to the side

Making Rescues Using a Body Board

Roll on rescue with an unconscious casualty

Ask your partner to pretend he is unconscious (tell the lifeguard what you are doing). Put his hand on the edge of the board (1). Roll it towards you once (2) and then again (3). Once your partner is on the board (4), swim around to the rear. Lie behind him and grab hold of each side of the board and kick to the side (5).

Swim and tow rescue

Paddle to your partner, dismount and offer the board. Tow her to safety using the board as a rescue aid.

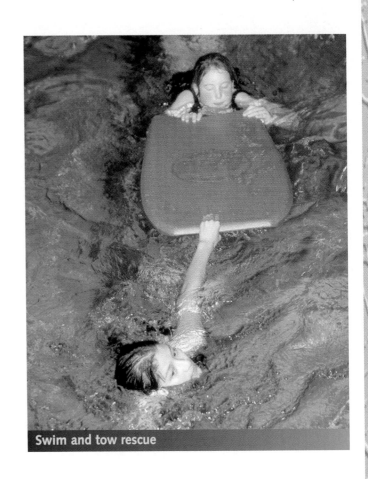

Swim and tow rescue

Give Rescue Breathing to an unconscious casualty
Ask your partner to pretend he is unconscious and paddle out to him. Slide off your board on the opposite side of your partner. Turn him so he is face up. Use his clothing or a chin grip to float him on to the side of the board, putting one hand under his armpit to secure him. Give Rescue Breathing. (See page 79.)

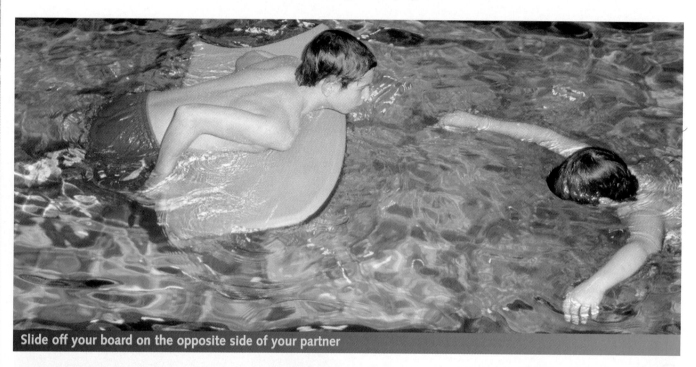

Slide off your board on the opposite side of your partner

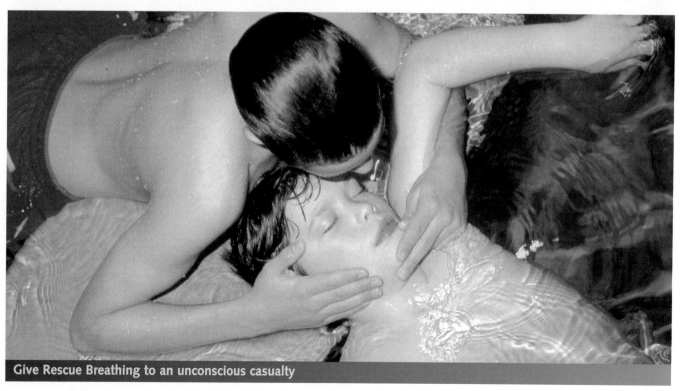

Give Rescue Breathing to an unconscious casualty

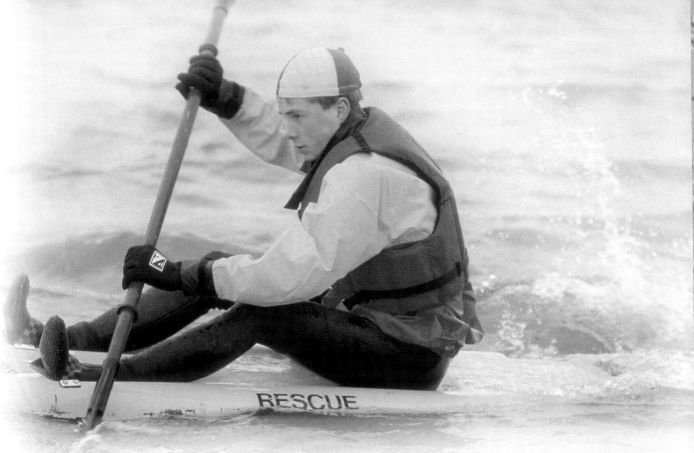

Using a Rescue Ski

Launching and paddling

Get into the water pushing the ski. Climb on to the ski in shallow water and sit with your feet in the straps. Paddle with the double ended paddle raising and lowering alternate ends and pull on the end in the water.

Rescuing a conscious casualty

Paddle out to the casualty and tell her to hold on to the back of the ski. Paddle back to safety.

Rescuing an unconscious casualty

Use the same way as for a body board.

Using a Rescue Board

Launching and paddling

Get into the water pushing the rescue board in front of you. Climb on to the board just behind the middle and lie down. To paddle the board you can kneel and paddle using Butterfly arms or lie flat on the board and use Front Crawl arms.

Butterfly arms

Move your arms just as you do in Front Crawl, but move them together.

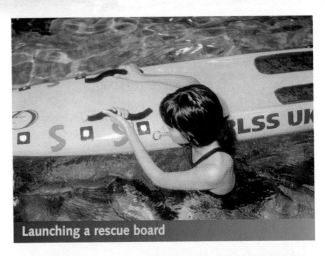

Launching a rescue board

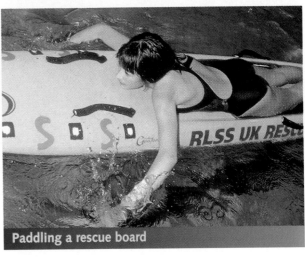

Paddling a rescue board

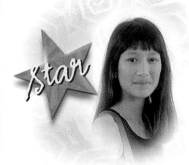

Rookie

*H*i, I'm Natasha and I have been a Rookie for 2 years. The best thing is knowing that I could rescue someone some day. I have been practising rescues with the rescue board and could use it if I saw anyone unconscious in the water.

Rescuing a conscious casualty

Grab your partner's wrist and slide off the rescue board on the opposite side (1). Stretch his arms across the board (2) and help him on to the board (3). Lie him on his front, climb on to the board behind him (4) and paddle to safety (5).

Rescuing an unconscious casualty

Use the same way as for a body board.

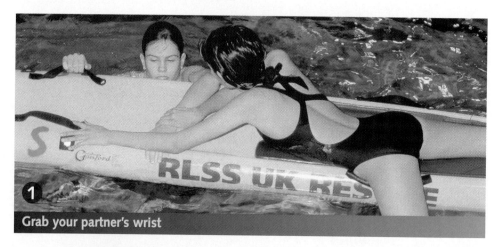

1 Grab your partner's wrist

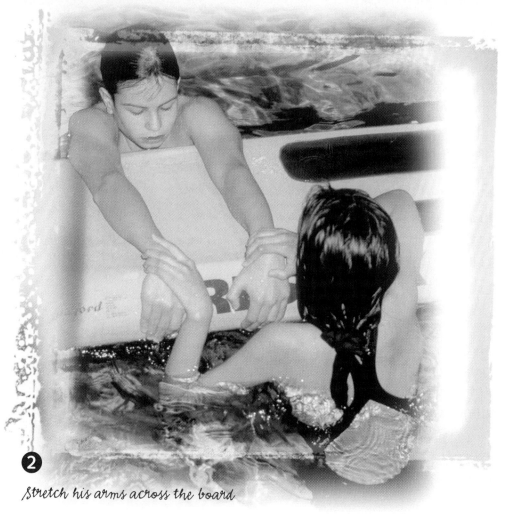

2 *Stretch his arms across the board*

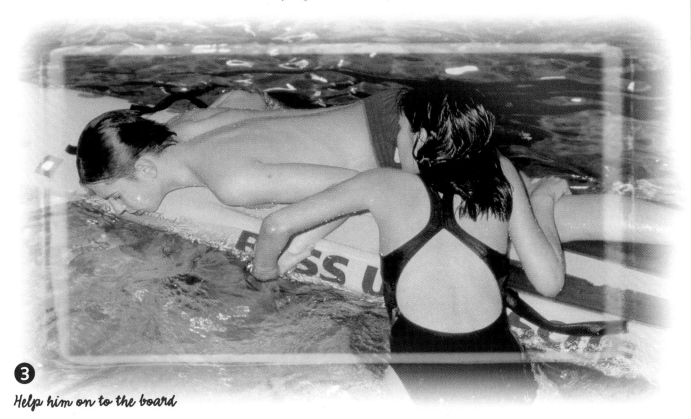

3

Help him on to the board

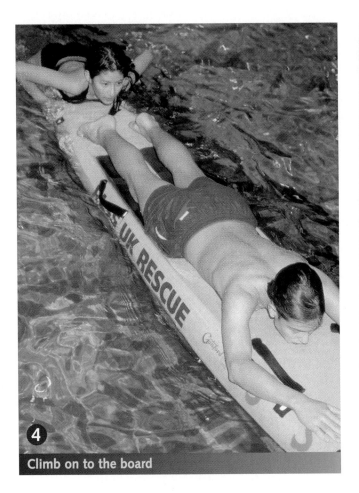

4

Climb on to the board

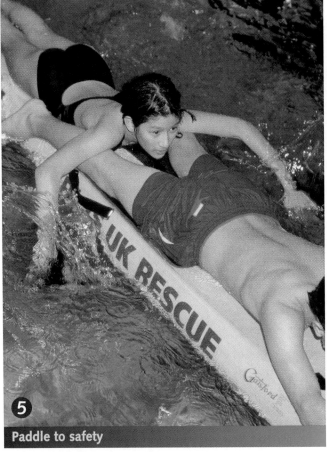

5

Paddle to safety

Aftercare Help given to a casualty by a rescuer, bystander or qualified doctor after an emergency.

Airway The passage between the mouth and the lungs.

Assessment Deciding what has happened and what to do.

Bends Types of knots.

Body Board A short lightweight board used for body-surfing and which can also be used as a rescue aid.

Body Language Signals that your body sends to other people.

Buoyancy Jacket A special jacket to keep you afloat in the water.

Butterfly Stroke A type of swimming stroke placing both arms in the water at the same time.

Cardiopulmonary Resuscitation (CPR) A combination of Rescue Breathing and chest compressions to keep a casualty alive when the heart has stopped beating.

Casualty An injured person or a person needing help.

Chest Compression Rhythmical pressing down on a casualty's chest to keep his blood circulating when his heart has stopped beating.

HM Coastguard The emergency service working at the coast.

Current Water moving in one direction.

Customer Relations The way a lifeguard deals with other people who use the swimming pool or beach.

Dolphin Kick Keeping your legs together and kicking both legs up and down in the water at the same time.

Dressing A bandage or something used to cover a wound.

Emergency Something which suddenly happens which demands immediate attention.

Emergency Response Action taken immediately to help a casualty and stop him from being injured any further.

Emergency Services Qualified people who help you in an emergency.

Epilepsy A disease of the nervous system causing fits.

Faint To feel so dizzy that everything goes black and you fall down.

Fins Special shoes shaped like paddles to make you swim faster.

First Aid The first treatment of an injury.

HELP Position (Heat Escape Lessening Posture) A survival position where you hold a floating object to save body heat if you fall into cold water.

Hitches Types of knots.

HUDDLE Position A survival position to save body heat in cold water for groups of two or more people.

Hygiene Keeping things clean so you can remain healthy and prevent disease.

Hypothermia When a body's inside temperature drops so much that it cannot heat itself up again without help.

Inshore Rescue Boat A rescue boat for use near to the shore.

International Distress Signal A signal recognised in every country where a person in difficulty in the water is waving one arm from side to side above their head to attract attention.

Jetty A small landing stage for boats.

Life Buoy A device that floats to support a person in the water.

Life Jacket A special jacket which will keep you afloat and keep you on your back in the water.

Lifeguard A qualified person whose job is to supervise safety and rescue people in pools and open water.

Lifesaver Someone who helps anyone in difficulty and cares for a casualty.

Life Support Keeping a casualty alive until help arrives.

Lock A section of a river or canal fitted with gates and sluices so that boats can be raised or lowered to the level beyond each gate.

Lock Keeper Someone who is responsible for the organisation and safety at a canal lock.

Mask Something you wear over your face when snorkelling to help you see underwater.

Open Water Any water found outside except for swimming pools.

Paddle Craft Any vessel or board moved through the water by paddling.

Paramedics Ambulance crew who are trained to keep you alive in an emergency using special equipment.

Patrol Zone Area patrolled by lifeguards.

Personal Floatation Device (PFD) A lifejacket or buoyancy jacket which you wear to keep you afloat in the water.

Pulse The throbbing that can be felt as the blood is pumped by the heart around the body.

Recovery Position The position an unconscious casualty is put in to aid recovery and to prevent obstruction of the airway.

Rescue Aid Anything used to help carry out a rescue.

Rescue Board A special surfboard which you paddle with your hands while kneeling or lying on it.

Rescue Breathing Where you blow air through a casualty's mouth or nose into his lungs to keep him alive.

Rescue Ski A rescue craft on which a rescuer sits and paddles with a single twin-bladed paddle.

Reservoir A place where a large amount of water is stored.

Resuscitation Another name for Rescue Breathing.

Resuscitation Manikin Model of a person used to practise Rescue Breathing and CPR techniques.

Scanning This is what a lifeguard does as he searches from side to side looking for people in difficulty in the water.

Self Rescue How to help your own rescue and survive in water.

Shock This is what happens when the brain and body do not get enough blood.

Snorkel Breathing tube for underwater swimming.

Sprain To twist your leg or arm so that it swells and is painful.

Stand-off Position A position where you stay out of reach of the casualty in the water.

Support Position A position where you support the casualty by the side in the water.

Surface Dive A dive from the surface of the water.

Tide The movement of the sea towards the land and away from the land.

Torpedo Buoy A rescue aid used by lifeguards.

Tow When a casualty is pulled through the water.

Tread Water Something you do to keep afloat and stationary in deep water.

Unconscious When the brain is not thinking and the body cannot move.

Water Safety Code A four point code to keep you safe near water.

Weir A small dam across a river or canal where fast flowing water is channelled.

If you have enjoyed learning how to use mask, snorkel and fins for your Rookie Snorkelling Certificate, you may decide that you would like to find out more about snorkelling or perhaps even learn sub-aqua diving.

Snorkelling with The British Sub-Aqua Club

If you would like to find out more, then contact the headquarters of The British Sub-Aqua Club (BSAC) who will put you in touch with the BSAC snorkelling and diving clubs in your area.

If you decide to continue snorkelling, your Rookie Snorkelling Certificate will count towards your BSAC Basic Snorkel Diver Award. You may need to take a test when you start with The British Sub-Aqua Club but you shouldn't find it difficult to pass because you will have had all the necessary training. You will also be able to buy a BSAC Basic Snorkel Diver Certificate and badge to add to your RLSS UK Rookie badges. If you want to start snorkelling with The British Sub-Aqua Club you should be 8 years old.

If you already have a BSAC Basic Snorkel Diver or BSAC Snorkel Diver qualification you can use this to get a Rookie Snorkelling Certificate when you join the Rookie programme.

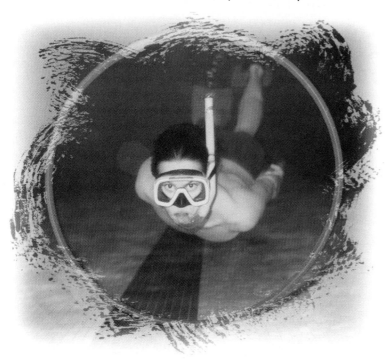

When you have achieved the BSAC Basic Snorkel Diver Award, you can progress to take the BSAC Snorkel Diver Award, the BSAC Open Water Snorkel Diver Award and BSAC Advanced Snorkel Diver Award.

You have to be 14 years old to start aqualung diving. Snorkelling is a good beginning to aqualung diving, so if you are not 14 yet, try and improve your snorkelling as much as you can.

You will find the address of BSAC Headquarters at the back of this book.

The Water Safety Code

A leaflet introducing the four point Water Safety Code
to young people.
Available from RLSS UK Enterprises Ltd.
Order code TP-WSC

"What Can I Do?" Junior Life Support Leaflet

Comic-style leaflet packed with information about what
to do in an emergency.
Available from RLSS UK Enterprises Ltd.

Rescue Breathing

Full colour comic-style leaflet on how to do Rescue Breathing.
Available from RLSS UK Enterprises Ltd.
Order Code TP-RBC

Beach Lifeguarding

Training Manual for the Beach Lifeguard covering beach
management, communication skills, drowning prevention,
emergency response and much more.
Available from RLSS UK Enterprises Ltd.
Order Code TP-BLG

Lifesaving

The complete book about lifesaving.
Available from RLSS UK Enterprises Ltd.
Order Code TP-LSH

Life Support

Essential reference book dealing with all aspects of
resuscitation and CPR.
Available from RLSS UK Enterprises Ltd.
Order Code TP-LSB

Pool Lifeguarding

Training manual for Pool Lifeguards.
Available from RLSS UK Enterprises Ltd.
Order Code TP-PLG

First Aid Manual

Produced by St John Ambulance, St Andrew's Ambulance
Association and the British Red Cross. Always use the latest edition.
Available from bookshops.

Index

Index